The Big
Dash Diet

Cookbook for Beginners

Low Sodium Recipes and 4 Weeks Meal Plan to Improve Your Health

Stephanie Bullard

Contents

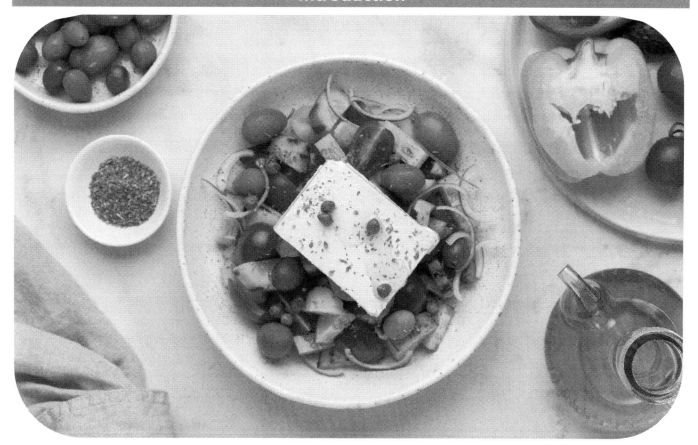

Good health is not merely down to genetics; it is something you need to maintain through your own efforts. Genetics do help, but not as much as your lifestyle and a healthy dietary approach. Even the healthiest young individual can experience difficulties in later life if they fail to keep active and fit.

It is not just how much food you consume that determines your level of nourishment—it is also the quality of that food. Some nutrients are necessary for the body, but excessive intake can cause imbalances, leading to various disorders. We see the results of this today. Sodium, for example, is a micronutrient or mineral that our bodies need a certain amount of for healthy functioning. However, our modern diet means that we regularly ingest excessive amounts of the mineral. Sodium has a considerable role to play in the control of blood pressure. People with hypertension are more sensitive to sodium intake, and high consumption can severely affect their blood pressure levels. Therefore, the Dash Diet encourages sodium intake to be kept under control.

So, if you have constantly been struggling with this health problem (or others), then this cookbook, with its 80 low-sodium recipes, and a 28-day meal plan, is definitely going to help you stay fit.

What is the Dash Diet?

The Dash Diet stands for "Dietary Approaches to Stop Hypertension." As its name suggests, the diet plan was created to regulate hypertension using a specific food pattern. The diet is not entirely vegetarian, as some may believe, but rather a well-balanced blend of essential nutrients. Low-fat dairy foods, fruits, whole grains, and vegetables make up the bulk of this diet. Experts at the National Heart, Lung, and Blood Institute of the United States first endorsed Dash as an optimum eating plan for preventing and minimizing hypertension by reducing fat and sodium intake.

The Dash Diet focuses on various goals regarding daily food intake. Everything is taken into consideration, from the type and form of the ingredients to the overall amount and per meal serving. The goal of such a program is to achieve a realistic nutritional balance. Before a person begins the Dash Diet, professionals will examine their eating habits, health status, metabolic rate, signs of illness, and fitness routine. From this, they will then create a road map to better health.

Advantages of the Dash Diet

Like many other dietary programs, Dash is health-oriented, with the primary goal of meeting specific goals for living a healthy lifestyle. These goals include the prevention of some diseases as well as the treatment of others. Though Dash is well-known for reducing hypertension effectively, it also has several other health benefits.

1. Reduced Hypertension

The sodium and salt content of Dash is minimal. As a result, it helps to decrease hypertension and maintain healthy blood pressure. Dietary changes under the

Dash guidelines are recommended for hypertensive patients.

2. Weight Loss

Although it was not initially intended to affect body weight, this healthy method can aid in preventing obesity. A well-balanced, nutritious diet is linked to a speedier metabolism and less fat buildup. Thus, by maintaining daily intake through this diet plan, obesity can be avoided without cutting out any specific items. It can be used by people who want to lose weight healthily while also getting speedy results.

3. Heart Health

A healthy heart is the result of a diet low in fat and high in complex carbohydrates. Cardiovascular disease is more widespread nowadays as the modern diet is higher in fats and carbohydrates and low in fiber. This imbalance causes blockages in the veins and arteries, creating heart problems and, potentially, heart attacks or strokes. The Dash Diet allows for a reduced, more controlled intake of all of these foods, hence helping to prevent heart-related disorders.

4. Osteoporosis Prevention

Unfortunately, this condition is widespread among women in their forties and fifties. Because it is high in potassium, calcium, and proteins, Dash helps to prevent osteoporosis. The Dash food plan can help maintain the body's calcium and potassium balance if it is followed consistently.

5. Healthy Kidneys

Following the Dash Diet is a well-known method for avoiding kidney stones, a common occurrence when eating high-sodium foods. Dash contains no extra minerals that could build up in the kidneys or cause dehydration. Furthermore, a vital balance of salt and potassium is required for blood purification for proper kidney function. This balance is maintained when salt consumption is reduced.

6. Helps Regulate Diabetes

A diet that is low in empty calories can assist in lowering the level of simple sugars in the blood, reducing the risk of diabetes. Insulin deficiency is a complication of type 2 diabetes. Insulin is a hormone that regulates blood sugar levels. Because Dash contains minimal sugar-based foods, it is incredibly beneficial to such patients.

7. Reduces Risk of Cancer

No treatment has been shown to be more effective than food support for cancer patients. Because the Dash Diet is high in vitamins, fiber, and antioxidants, it helps prevent cancer from spreading throughout the body.

Foods Allowed on the Dash Diet

On a Dash Diet, it's safe to say that any food can be enjoyed as long as a balance is maintained. On a larger scale, this diet plan does not prohibit the consumption of most foods, but it does limit their quantity. The following is a list of foods that can be eaten on the Dash Diet:

1. Grains.
2. Vegetables.
3. Fruits.
4. Seeds
5. Nuts
6. Low-fat or no-fat dairy products
7. Beef and pork
8. Poultry
9. Seafood

Foods to Avoid on the Dash Diet

The Dash Diet forbids foods that can promote high blood pressure, hypertension, high blood sugar levels, and obesity. The following items should be consumed in smaller quantities:

1. Salt
2. Sugary beverages
3. Salted nuts
4. High-fat dairy products
5. Processed foods
6. Excessive animal-based fats

Tasty Cucumber, Celery, and Matcha Green Smoothie

Prep Time: 5 minutes
Cook Time: 5 minutes
Serves: 1
Ingredients
- ½cupcashew milk
- 1baby cucumber
- 1celery stalk
- ½avocado
- 1tbsp.coconut oil or MCT oil
- 1tsp.matcha powder
- Sweetener of choice,to taste

Preparation
1. In a blender, combine all of the ingredients and blend until smooth.
Serving Suggestion: Serve with chopped almonds or walnuts sprinkled on top.
Variation Tip: Spinach can be added for added flavor.
Nutritional Information Per Serving:
Calories 278 | Protein 3g | Carbohydrate 12g | Dietary fiber 3g | Sugar 0g | Fat 27g | Sodium 35mg

Carrot & Turmeric Smoothie

Prep Time: 35 minutes
Cook Time: 0 minutes
Serves: 2
Ingredients:
The Juice:
- 2 cups carrots
- 1.5 cups filtered water
The Smoothie:
- 1 large + more for sweetness as desired ripe banana
- 1 cup frozen or fresh pineapple
- ½ tablespoon fresh ginger
- ½ cup carrot juice
- ¼ teaspoon ground turmeric
- ½ teaspoon cinnamon
- 1 tablespoon lime juice
- 1 cup unsweetened almond milk
Preparation:
1. Add the water and carrots to the blender. Pulse until smooth.
2. Add more water as needed, scraping down its sides.
3. Strain and discard the pulp.
4. Keep the juice in the refrigerator for 30 minutes.
5. Toss the rest of the fixings into the blender for the smoothie and mix thoroughly.
6. Add in the carrot juice and pulse some more
7. Serve in two chilled glasses.
Serving Suggestion: Serve with a sprinkle of ground turmeric.
Variation Tip: You can substitute the almond milk with coconut milk.
Nutritional Information per Serving:
Calories 144 | Fat 2.3 g | Sodium 112 mg | Carbs 32 g | Fiber5 g | Sugar 17.5 g | Protein 2.4 g

Kiwi Clementine Smoothie

Prep Time: 10 minutes
Cook Time: 0 minutes
Serves: 2
Ingredients:
- 2 kiwis, peeled and diced
- 2 clementines, peeled and diced
- 1 banana, peeled and sliced
- 1 cup coconut water
- 2 cups baby spinach
- ¼ cup Greek yogurt
Preparation:
1. Ready all the fruits and vegetables, then put them in a blender.
2. Toss in the rest of the smoothie ingredients.
3. Hit the pulse button to blend the smoothie until smooth.
4. Chill the smoothie for 2 hours in the refrigerator.
5. Serve chilled and fresh.
Serving Suggestion: Serve the smoothie with cranberry scones.
Variation Tip: Add chocolate chips to the smoothie.
Nutritional Information per Serving:
Calories 182 | Fat 1.6g |Sodium 161mg | Carbs 40.1g | Fiber 7.1g | Sugar 25.1g | Protein 6.4g

Blackberry Smoothie

Prep Time: 5 minutes
Servings: 1
Ingredients:
• 1 cup frozen blueberries
• ½ cup almond milk
• ½ banana, sliced
• ½ cup crushed ice
Preparation:
1. Add the blackberries, almond milk, and banana slices to a high-speed blender and blend well.
2. Pour into serving glasses and top with crushed ice.
3. Serve and enjoy!
Serving Suggestion: Top with blackberries before serving.
Variation Tip: You can use any sweetener of your choice.
Nutritional Information per Serving:
Calories: 412|Fat: 29.3g|Sat Fat: 25.4g|Carbohydrates: 41.1g |Fiber: 7.7g|Sugar: 25.6g|Protein: 4.5g

Strawberry and Oat Smoothie

Prep Time: 20 minutes
Servings: 4
Ingredients:
• ½ cup rolled oats

• ½ banana, peeled and sliced
• 1¼ cups unsweetened almond milk
• ½ cup strawberries, peeled, sectioned, and seeded
• ½ cup ice cubes
Preparation:
1. Put the rolled oats into a high-speed blender and pulse until they're completely chopped.
2. Add the banana slices, almond milk, and orange. Pulse to form a smooth mixture.
3. Pour the mixture into two serving glasses and add a few ice cubes.
4. Serve and enjoy!
Serving Suggestion: Serve with the chopped strawberries on top.
Variation Tip: You can replace strawberries with raspberries.
Nutritional Information per Serving:
Calories: 202|Fat: 6.4g|Sat Fat: 0.7g|Carbohydrates: 34.1g|Fiber: 6.4g|Sugar: 12.4g|Protein: 5.3g

Avocado and Spinach Smoothie

Prep Time: 15 minutes
Servings: 4
Ingredients:
• 1 tablespoon hemp seeds
• 2 cups fresh baby spinach
• 3–4 drops liquid stevia
• ½ teaspoon ground cinnamon
• ½ avocado, peeled, pitted, and chopped
• 2 cups filtered water, chilled
Preparation:
1. Add the baby spinach and avocado with all other ingredients in a high-speed blender.
2. Blend until a smooth mixture forms, then pour into serving glasses.
3. Serve and enjoy!
Serving Suggestion: Serve with hemp seeds on top.
Variation Tip: Crushed ice can also be added.
Nutritional Information per Serving:
Calories: 132|Fat: 11.7g|Sat Fat: 1.2g|Carbohydrates: 6.1g|Fiber: 4.5g|Sugar: 0.4g|Protein: 3.1g

Cucumber and Kiwi Smoothie

Prep Time: 5 minutes
Serves: 1
Ingredients:

- 1 kiwi, peeled and chopped
- 1 drop liquid stevia
- ½ cucumber, peeled and sliced
- 1 cup water
- 1 tablespoon cilantro leaves
- ¼ tablespoon ginger, peeled and chopped

Preparation:
1. Add kiwi, stevia, cucumber, water, cilantro and ginger in a high-speed blender.
2. Blend until a smooth mixture is formed and pour in serving glasses.
3. Serve and enjoy!
Serving Suggestions: Top it with crushed ice.
Variation Tip: Ginger can be omitted.
Nutritional Information per Serving:
Calories: 74 | Fat: 0.7g | Sat Fat: 0.1g | Carbohydrates: 17.6g | Fiber: 3.2g | Sugar: 9.4g | Protein: 2g

Apple and Pear Smoothie

Prep Time: 10 minutes
Serves: 4
Ingredients:
- 4 apples, peeled and chopped
- 4 cups mustard greens, chopped
- 4 pears, peeled, cored and chopped
- ½ teaspoon ground cinnamon
- 3 cups water
- ½ cup ice cubes
Preparation:
1. Add everything in a high-speed blender and blend until smooth.
2. Pour in serving glasses and serve with a smile.
Serving Suggestions: Top with whipped cream before serving.
Variation Tip: You can also use coconut sugar to enhance taste.
Nutritional Information per Serving:
Calories: 272 | Fat: 2.3g | Sat Fat: 1.4g | Carbohydrates: 67g | Fiber: 13.9g | Sugar: 45.9g | Protein: 3.1g

Pomegranate Green Smoothie

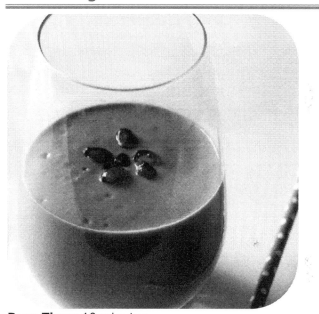

Prep Time: 10 minutes
Cook Time: 0 minutes
Serves: 2
Ingredients:
- 7 ounces pomegranate juice
- 1 apple, sliced
- 2 cups spinach or kale
- 1 banana, peeled and chopped
Preparation:
1. Ready all the fruits and put them in a blender.
2. Toss in the rest of the smoothie ingredients.
3. Hit the pulse button to blend the smoothie until smooth.
4. Chill the smoothie for 2 hours in the refrigerator.
5. Serve chilled and fresh.
Serving Suggestion: Serve the smoothie with cranberry scones.
Variation Tip: Add crushed walnuts or pecans to the smoothie.
Nutritional Information per Serving:
Calories 195 | Fat 3g |Sodium 55mg | Carbs 17g | Fiber 1g | Sugar 25g | Protein 1g

Mango Smoothie

Prep Time: 10 minutes
Serves: 4
Ingredients:
- 4 mangoes, peeled and chopped
- 1 teaspoon organic vanilla extract
- 3 cups fat-free milk
- 2 bananas, peeled and sliced
- 4 tablespoons chopped almonds

Preparation:
1. Add mangoes, vanilla extract, fat-free milk, bananas and almonds in a blender and blend properly.
2. Pour in serving glasses and serve with a smile.

Serving Suggestions: Top with mango slices before serving.
Variation Tip: Almonds can be omitted.
Nutritional Information per Serving:
Calories: 359 | Fat: 4.4g | Sat Fat: 0.6g | Carbohydrates: 74.2g | Fiber: 7.7g | Sugar: 62.5g | Protein: 10.7g

Kiwi Peach Smoothie

Prep Time: 10 minutes
Cook Time: 0 minutes
Serves: 2
Ingredients:
- 3 handfuls leafy greens
- 2 kiwis, peeled
- 1½ cups peach, peeled and cubed
- 1½ banana, frozen
- 1½ tablespoons chia seeds
- 1 cup almond milk
- 3 ice cubes

Preparation:
1. Ready all the fruits and vegetables, then put them in a blender.
2. Toss in the rest of the smoothie ingredients.
3. Hit the pulse button to blend the smoothie until smooth.
4. Chill the smoothie for 2 hours in the refrigerator.
5. Serve chilled and fresh.

Serving Suggestion: Serve the smoothie with cranberry muffins.
Variation Tip: Add a drizzle of maple syrup on top.
Nutritional Information per Serving:
Calories 250 | Fat 10g | Sodium 118mg | Carbs 52g | Fiber 10.2g | Sugar 30g | Protein 6.8g

High-Protein Strawberry Smoothie

Prep Time: 10 minutes
Cook Time: 10 minutes
Serves: 1
Ingredients
- ½ cup low salt, low-fat cottage cheese
- ¾ cup 1% milk
- 1 cup fresh or frozen strawberries (you can sub this with a banana or ½ cup of another berry or sliced mangoes)

Preparation
1. Add all ingredients, in order, to a blender or Nutribullet.
2. Blend until smooth.
3. Pour into a tall glass and enjoy!

Serving Suggestion: Add fresh fruit to the glass as garnish and serve for breakfast.
Variation Tip: You can use any fruit you like in place of the strawberries, but berries (such as blueberries and raspberries) or bananas pair best with cottage cheese. You can also use half a banana with ½ cup of strawberries.
Nutritional Information Per Serving:
Calories 215 | Protein 22g | Carbohydrates 26g | Dietary Fiber 3g | Sugar 21g | Fat 2.8g | Sodium 141mg

Delicious Cinnamon Almond Keto Shake

Prep Time: 5 minutes
Cook Time: 5 minutes
Serves: 1
Ingredients
- 1cupcoffee
- 4coconut milk ice cubes,or ⅓ to ½ cup coconut milk
- 1tbsp.coconut oil or MCT oil
- 2tbsp.almond butter
- 1tbsp.flax seeds
- ½tspcinnamon
- Sweetener of choice,to taste
- Pinchof salt

Preparation
1. In a blender, combine all of the ingredients and blend until smooth.
2. Serve and enjoy!
Serving Suggestion: Serve as a delicious snack.
Variation Tip: Add honey for added flavor.
Nutritional Information Per Serving:
Calories 503 | Protein 9g | Carbohydrate 11g | Dietary Fiber 2g | Sugar 0g | Fat 49g | Sodium 55mg

Watermelon-Cranberry Agua Fresca

Prep Time: 5 minutes
Cook Time: 5 minutes
Serves: 4
Ingredients
- 2½ lbs. seedless watermelon, rind removed and diced (about 7 cups)
- 1 cup fruit-sweetened cranberry juice (sometimes called cranberry nectar)

- ¼ cup fresh lime juice
- 1 lime, cut into 6 slices
Preparation
1. Place the melon in a blender or food processor. Process until smooth.
2. Pass the puree through a fine-mesh sieve placed over a bowl to eliminate the pulp and clarify the juice.
3. Pour the juice into a large pitcher. Add the cranberry and lime juices and stir to combine.
Serving Suggestion: Refrigerate until very cold. Pour into tall chilled glasses and garnish each with a slice of lime.
Variation Tip: Aguas frescas are popular fresh-fruit drinks in Mexico. Although water is a standard ingredient, this undiluted version is the perfect thirst quencher.
Nutritional Information Per Serving:
Calories 84 | Protein 1g | Carbohydrate 20g | Dietary fiber 1g | Sugar 0g | Fat 0g | Sodium 9mg

Green Smoothie

Prep Time: 5 minutes
Cook Time: 5 minutes
Serves: 4
Ingredients
- 1 banana
- Juice of 1 lemon (about 4 tbsp.)
- ½ cup strawberries
- ½ cup other berries, such as blackberries or blueberries
- 2 oz. fresh raw baby spinach (about 2 cups)
- Fresh mint to taste
- 1 cup cold water or ice
Preparation
1. Place all ingredients in a blender or juicer and puree.
2. Enjoy!
Serving Suggestion: Serve for breakfast or as a snack.
Variation Tip: Cardamom can be added to enhance the taste.
Nutritional Information Per Serving:
Calories 64 | Protein 0.5g | Carbohydrate 12g | Dietary fiber 2g | Sugar 0g | Fat 0g | Sodium 15mg

Psyllium Kale Smoothie

Prep Time: 10 minutes
Cook Time: 0 minutes
Serves: 2
Ingredients:
- 1 cup coconut water
- 1 banana, peeled and sliced
- 1 handful kale, chopped
- 1 cup pineapple chunks
- 1 teaspoon psyllium husk
- ½ teaspoon spirulina powder

Preparation:
1. Ready all the fruits and vegetables, then put them in a blender.
2. Toss in the rest of the smoothie ingredients.
3. Hit the pulse button to blend the smoothie until smooth.
4. Chill the smoothie for 2 hours in the refrigerator.
5. Serve chilled and fresh.

Serving Suggestion: Serve the smoothie with cranberry scones.
Variation Tip: Add crushed cashews on top.
Nutritional Information per Serving:
Calories 149 | Fat 1g |Sodium 8mg | Carbs 16g | Fiber 0.8g | Sugar 56g | Protein 1g

Grapes and Kale Smoothie

Prep Time: 10 minutes
Serves: 4
Ingredients:

- 4 cups fresh kale, chopped
- 2 cups seedless green grapes
- 3 cups water

- ½ cup ice cubes
- 4 drops stevia
- 2 tablespoons fresh lime juice

Preparation:
1. Add everything in a food processor and pulse until smooth.
2. Pour in serving glasses and serve with a smile.

Serving Suggestions: Top with crushed ice before serving.
Variation Tip: You can omit stevia.

Nutritional Information per Serving:
Calories: 91 | Fat: 0g | Sat Fat: 0g | Carbohydrates: 22.7g | Fiber: 1.6g| Sugar: 11.9g | Protein: 2.6g

Cucumber and Greens Smoothie

Prep Time: 10 minutes
Servings: 2
Ingredients:
- ½ cup lettuce, torn
- 1 small cucumber, peeled and chopped
- ¼ cup fresh mint leaves
- ¼ cup ice cubes
- ¼ cup fresh parsley leaves
- 1½ cups filtered water
- 1 teaspoon fresh lemon juice
- 2 cups mixed fresh greens
- 2–3 drops liquid stevia

Preparation:
1. Put the cucumber with all the other ingredients in a high-speed blender.
2. Blend until a smooth mixture forms, then pour into serving glasses.
3. Serve and enjoy!

Serving Suggestion: Top the drinks with crushed ice.
Variation Tip: Lemon juice can be replaced with lime juice.
Nutritional Information per Serving:
Calories: 50|Fat: 0.5g|Sat Fat: 0g|Carbohydrates: 11.3g|Fiber: 3.6g|Sugar: 3.2g|Protein: 2.5g

Kale and Apple Smoothie

Prep Time: 10 minutes
Serves: 4
Ingredients:
- 4 cups fresh baby kale
- 2 tablespoons chia seeds
- 4 cups water
- 2 bananas, sliced
- 2 apples, peeled and chopped

Preparation:

1. Add everything in a high-speed blender and blend until a smooth mixture is formed.
2. Pour in serving glasses and serve.
Serving Suggestions: Serve with apple slices on the top.
Variation Tip: You can add dates to enhance taste.
Nutritional Information per Serving:
Calories: 168 | Fat: 2.9g | Sat Fat: 0.1g |
Carbohydrates: 36.9g | Fiber: 8.2g | Sugar: 18.8g |
Protein: 3.9g

Cantaloupe Smoothie

Prep Time: 5 minutes
Cook Time: 5 minutes
Serves: 2
Ingredients
- ½ cupnon-fat or low-fat milk
- 1frozen banana, sliced
- 5.3 oz. non-fat vanilla Greek yogurt
- ½ cupice

- 1 tsp.honey
- 2½ cupscubed frozen cantaloupe, peeled and cubed
Preparation:
1. Place the milk, banana, yogurt, ice, and honey in a blender and process until smooth.
2. Add the cantaloupe pieces and process until smooth.
3. Serve immediately.
Serving Suggestion: Serve the smoothie as a snack topped with fruit.
Variation Tip: An economical and healthy way to add protein to smoothies, soups, and other recipes is to add a couple of tablespoons of non-fat dry milk powder to the ingredients. Non-fat dry milk powder has all of fluid non-fat milk's nutritional attributes, only in powdered form. If you don't drink much milk and are afraid of spoilage, consider adding dry milk to your pantry staples.
Nutritional Information Per Serving:
Calories 214 | Protein 11g | Carbohydrate 46g |
Dietary Fiber 3g | Sugar 18g | Fat 1g | Sodium 14mg

Banana Smoothie

Prep Time: 10 minutes
Serves: 4
Ingredients:
- 4 bananas, peeled and sliced
- 1 teaspoon organic vanilla extract
- ½ teaspoon ground cinnamon
- 3 cups unsweetened almond milk
Preparation:
1. Add bananas, vanilla extract, cinnamon and almond milk in a blender.
2. Blend well until a firm mixture is formed.
3. Pour in serving glasses and serve.
Serving Suggestions: Serve with banana slices on the top.
Variation Tip: Crushed ice can also be added in the smoothie.
Nutritional Information per Serving:
Calories: 139 | Fat: 3g |Sat Fat: 0.4g |
Carbohydrates: 28.8g | Fiber: 4g | Sugar: 14.6g
|Protein: 2.1g

Pear Smoothie

Prep Time: 10 minutes
Servings: 4
Ingredients:
- 1 teaspoon organic vanilla extract
- 4 pears, peeled and chopped
- 3 cups milk, fat-free
- 4 tablespoons almonds, chopped
- 2 bananas, peeled and sliced

Preparation:
1. Add all the ingredients to a blender and blend thoroughly.
2. Pour into serving glasses and serve with a smile.

Serving Suggestion: Top with pear slices before serving.
Variation Tip: Almonds can be omitted.
Nutritional Information per Serving:
Calories: 359|Fat: 4.4g|Sat Fat: 0.6g|Carbohydrates: 74.2g|Fiber: 7.7g|Sugar: 62.5g|Protein: 10.7g

Cucumber Medjool Smoothie

Prep Time: 10 minutes
Cook Time: 0 minutes
Serves: 2
Ingredients:
- 1 cup water
- ½ cucumber, peeled and cubed
- 1 frozen banana, peeled and sliced
- 1 cup mixed berries, frozen
- 1 teaspoon spirulina powder
- 1 Medjool date pitted
- 1 handful baby spinach

Preparation:
1. Ready all the fruits and vegetables, then put them in a blender.
2. Toss in the rest of the smoothie ingredients.

3. Hit the pulse button to blend the smoothie until smooth.
4. Chill the smoothie for 2 hours in the refrigerator.
5. Serve chilled and fresh.
Serving Suggestion: Serve the smoothie with banana bread.
Variation Tip: Add chopped nuts to the smoothie
Nutritional Information per Serving:
Calories 165 | Fat 0.6g |Sodium 95mg | Carbs 34g | Fiber 7.3g | Sugar 10g | Protein 3.8g

High-Calorie, High-Protein Smoothie (Lactose-Free)

Prep Time: 5 minutes
Cook Time: 5 minutes
Serves: 1
Ingredients
- 1 cup soy yogurt
- 1 cup vanilla soy milk
- 1 medium banana, cut into chunks
- 2 tbsp. wheat germ
- 2 tbsp. protein powder

Preparation
1. Combine the yogurt, soy milk, banana chunks, wheat germ, and protein powder in a blender. Blend until smooth.
Serving Suggestion: Pour into a tall chilled glass and serve immediately.
Variation Tip: To make the recipe higher in calories, add 1 tbsp. of flaxseed oil for an additional 120 calories, 14 grams of fat, and no added sodium or cholesterol.
Nutritional Information Per Serving:
Calories 519 | Protein 37g | Carbohydrate 77g | Dietary fiber 9g | Sugar 5g | Fat 7g | Sodium 472mg

16

Orange and Oat Smoothie

Prep Time: 5 minutes
Serves: 2
Ingredients:
- ½ cup rolled oats
- ½ banana, peeled and sliced
- 1¼ cups unsweetened almond milk
- 1 orange, peeled, sectioned and seeded
- ½ cup ice cubes

Preparation:
1. Add rolled oats in a high-speed blender and pulse until they are completely chopped.
2. Add in banana slices, almond milk and orange. Pulse to form a smooth mixture.
3. Pour in two serving glasses and add ice cubes in them.
4. Serve and enjoy!

Serving Suggestions: Serve with whipped cream on the top.
Variation Tip: Crushed ice can also be added.
Nutritional Information per Serving:
Calories: 202 | Fat: 6.4g | Sat Fat: 0.7g |
Carbohydrates: 34.1g | Fiber: 6.4g | Sugar: 12.4g |
Protein: 5.3g

Spirulina Smoothie

Prep Time: 10 minutes
Cook Time: 0 minutes
Serves: 2
Ingredients:
- 1 handful spinach
- 2 kiwi fruits, peeled
- 1 cup mango chunks
- ½ cup fresh orange juice
- 1 teaspoon spirulina powder

- 3 tablespoons unsweetened vanilla powder
Preparation:
1. Ready all the fruits and vegetables, then put them in a blender.
2. Toss in the rest of the smoothie ingredients.
3. Hit the pulse button to blend the smoothie until smooth.
4. Chill the smoothie for 2 hours in the refrigerator.
5. Serve chilled and fresh.
Serving Suggestion: Serve the smoothie with pumpkin tea cake.
Variation Tip: Add crushed walnuts or pecans on top.
Nutritional Information per Serving:
Calories 203 | Fat 8.9g |Sodium 50mg | Carbs 22g |
Fiber 1.2g | Sugar 11.3g | Protein 5.3g

Strawberry Smoothie

Prep Time: 5 minutes
Serves: 1
Ingredients:
- ½ cup fresh strawberries, sliced
- 1 tablespoon unsalted almonds
- ¾ cup fat-free milk
- ½ banana, sliced

Preparation:
1. Add everything in a blender and blend until a firm mixture is formed.
2. Take out and pour in serving glasses.
3. Serve and enjoy!
Serving Suggestions: Top with strawberry sliced before serving.
Variation Tip: You can add organic vanilla essence to enhance taste.
Nutritional Information per Serving:
Calories: 177 | Fat: 3.4g | Sat Fat: 0.3 |
Carbohydrates: 29.3g | Fiber: 3.7g | Sugar: 20g |
Protein: 8.4g

Orange Dream Smoothie

Prep Time: 8 minutes
Cook Time: 8 minutes
Serves: 4
Ingredients
- 1½ cups orange juice, chilled
- 1 cup light vanilla soy milk, chilled
- ⅓ cup silken or soft tofu
- 1 tbsp. dark honey
- 1 tsp. grated orange zest
- ½ tsp. vanilla extract
- 5 ice cubes
- 4 peeled orange segments (about half an orange)

Preparation
1. Combine the orange juice, soy milk, tofu, honey, orange zest, vanilla, and ice cubes in a blender.
2. Blend until smooth and frothy, about 30 seconds.

Serving Suggestion: Pour into tall, chilled glasses and garnish each glass with an orange segment.
Variation Tip: For best results, use ice-cold soy milk and freshly squeezed orange juice.
Nutritional Information Per Serving:
Calories 101 | Protein 3g | Carbohydrate 20g | Dietary fiber 1g | Sugar 4g | Fat 1g | Sodium 40mg

Chocolaty Avocado Smoothie

Prep Time: 10 minutes
Servings: 2
Ingredients:
- ½ teaspoon organic vanilla extract
- 1 medium avocado, peeled, pitted, and chopped
- ¼ cup ice cubes
- 3 tablespoons cacao powder
- 1 small banana, peeled and sliced
- 1¾ cups fat-free milk, chilled

Preparation:
1. Put the cacao powder, avocado, and all the other ingredients in a high-speed blender.
2. Blend until a smooth mixture forms, then pour into serving glasses.
3. Serve and enjoy!

Serving Suggestion: Top with crushed ice before serving.
Variation Tip: You can also use almond milk.
Nutritional Information per Serving:
Calories: 358|Fat: 21.3g|Sat Fat: 3.4g|Carbohydrates: 36.5g|Fiber: 10g|Sugar: 18.4g|Protein: 11g

Fresh Fruit Smoothie

Prep Time: 5 minutes
Cook Time: 5 minutes
Serves: 4
Ingredients
- 1 cup fresh pineapple chunks
- ½ cup cantaloupe or other melon
- 1 cup fresh strawberries
- Juice of 2 oranges
- 1 cup cold water
- 1 tbsp. honey

Preparation
1. Remove the rind from pineapple and melon. Cut into chunks.
2. Remove the stems from the strawberries.
3. Place all ingredients in a blender and puree until smooth.

Serving Suggestion: Serve cold.
Variation Tip: You can prepare the ingredients ahead of time and store them in the refrigerator until you're ready to blend them.
Nutritional Information Per Serving:
Calories 72 | Protein 1g | Carbohydrate 17g | Dietary fiber 1g | Sugar 4g | Fat 0g | Sodium 7mg

Carrot and Orange Smoothie

Prep Time: 10 minutes
Servings: 2
Ingredients:
- 2 oranges, peeled and seeded
- 2 celery stalks, chopped
- 1½ cups ice
- 1 large carrot, peeled and sliced
- ¼ teaspoon fresh ginger, peeled

Preparation:
1. Place all the ingredients into a high-speed blender.
2. Blend until a smooth mixture forms, then pour into serving glasses.
3. Serve and enjoy!

Serving Suggestion: Serve with whipped cream on top.
Variation Tip: Crushed ice can also be added.
Nutritional Information per Serving:
Calories: 103|Fat: 0.3g|Sat Fat: 0g|Carbohydrates: 25g|Fiber: 5.5g|Sugar: 18.3g|Protein: 2.1g

Coconut Spirulina Smoothie

Prep Time: 10 minutes
Cook Time: 0 minutes
Serves: 2
Ingredients:
- 3 tablespoons coconut cream
- 1 small avocado, peeled, pitted and cubed
- 1 tablespoon grated ginger root
- 1 small orange, peeled diced

- 2 tablespoons maple syrup
- ½ teaspoon cinnamon powder
- 1 pinch cardamom spice
- 14 ounces coconut milk
- 1 scoop spirulina powder

Preparation:
1. Ready all the fruits and vegetables then put them in a blender.
2. Toss in the rest of the smoothie ingredients.
3. Hit the pulse button to blend the smoothie until smooth.
4. Chill the smoothie for 2 hours in the refrigerator.
5. Serve chilled and fresh.

Serving Suggestion: Serve the smoothie with cranberry muffins.
Variation Tip: Add crushed walnuts or pecans to the smoothie.
Nutritional Information per Serving:
Calories 258 | Fat 17g |Sodium 30mg | Carbs 26g | Fiber 10.2g | Sugar 11.4g | Protein 4.9g

Mixed Berries Smoothie

Prep Time: 10 minutes
Serves: 4
Ingredients:
- 2 cups fresh strawberries, hulled
- ½ cup raspberries
- 2 cups orange juice
- ½ cup fresh blackberries
- 1 cup ice cubes

Preparation:
1. In a high-speed blender, ad strawberries, raspberries, blackberries and orange juice. Blend well.
2. Pour in serving glasses and top with ice cubes.
3. Serve and enjoy!

Serving Suggestions: Serve with blackberries on the top.
Variation Tip: Blueberry syrup can be added to enhance taste.
Nutritional Information per Serving:
Calories: 95 | Fat: 0.7g | Sat Fat: 0.1g | Carbohydrates: 22g | Fiber: 3.6g | Sugar: 15.5g | Protein: 1.8g

Peach Avocado Smoothie

Prep Time: 5 minutes
Cook Time: 0 minutes
Serves: 2
Ingredients:
- 1½ cups frozen peaches
- 1½ cups nonfat milk
- 1 cup nonfat plain or vanilla Greek yogurt
- 1 avocado, peeled and pitted
- 1 tablespoon ground flaxseed
- 1½ teaspoons granulated stevia
- 1 teaspoon pure vanilla extract
- 2 cups ice cubes

Preparation:
1. Combine all the ingredients in a blender.
2. Purée until smooth.
3. Serve immediately.

Serving Suggestion: Garnish with peach slices.
Variation Tip: Feel free to use a no-calorie sweetener of your choice.
Nutritional Information per Serving:
Calories 323 | Fat 15g | Sodium 142mg | Carbs 32g | Fiber8g | Sugar 60g | Protein 21g

Green Veggie Smoothie

Prep Time: 10 minutes
Servings: 2
Ingredients:
- ½ green bell pepper, seeded and chopped
- 1 cup fresh spinach
- 2 cups filtered water, chilled
- ¼ cup green cabbage, chopped
- ¼ cup broccoli florets, chopped
- 3–4 drops liquid stevia

Preparation:
1. Add the broccoli with all the other ingredients to a high-speed blender.
2. Blend until a smooth mixture forms, then pour into serving glasses.
3. Serve and enjoy!

Serving Suggestion: Top with whipped cream before serving.
Variation Tip: You can also use coconut sugar to enhance the taste.
Nutritional Information per Serving:
Calories: 132|Fat: 11.7g|Sat Fat: 3g|Carbohydrates: 6.1g|Fiber: 0.4g|Sugar: 0g|Protein: 0.4g

Blueberry Smoothie

Prep Time: 5 minutes
Serves: 1
Ingredients:
- 1 cup frozen blueberries
- ½ cup almond milk
- ½ banana, sliced
- ½ cup crushed ice

Preparation:
4. Add blueberries, almond milk and banana slices in a high-speed blender and blend well.
5. Pour in serving glasses and top with crushed ice.
6. Serve and enjoy!

Serving Suggestions: Top with blueberries before serving.
Variation Tip: You can use any sweetener of your choice.
Nutritional Information per Serving:
Calories: 412 | Fat: 29.3g | Sat Fat: 25.4g | Carbohydrates: 41.1g | Fiber: 7.7g | Sugar: 25.6g | Protein: 4.5g

Pumpkin Smoothie

Prep Time: 10 minutes
Servings: 2
Ingredients:
- 1 cup homemade pumpkin puree
- 1 teaspoon ground flaxseeds
- 1½ cups unsweetened almond milk
- 1 medium banana, peeled and sliced
- ¼ teaspoon ground cinnamon
- ¼ cup ice cubes

Preparation:
1. Place the pumpkin puree, flaxseeds, banana, cinnamon, almond milk, and ice cubes in a blender.
2. Blend well until a smooth mixture forms.
3. Pour into serving glasses and serve.

Serving Suggestion: Serve with shaved coconut on top.
Variation Tip: Crushed ice can also be added to the smoothie.
Nutritional Information per Serving:
Calories: 264|Fat: 11.6g|Sat Fat: 1.1g|Carbohydrates: 16g|Fiber: 0g|Sugar: 0g|Protein: 10.6g

Golden Milk Smoothie

Prep Time: 5 minutes
Cook Time: 5 minutes
Serves: 1
Ingredients
- 8coconut milk ice cubes,thawed slightly (or 1 cup coconut milk)
- 2tbsp.additional coconut milk or water

- ½tspvanilla
- 1tbsp.coconut oil or MCT oil
- ½tspturmeric
- ¼tspcinnamon
- Pinchof ground ginger
- Pinchof salt
- Sweetener of choice,to taste

Preparation
1. In a blender, combine all of the ingredients and blend until smooth.

To make coconut milk ice cubes:
1. Shake the coconut milk can, blend the milk, or whisk until smooth and clump-free.
2. Freeze for 3-4 hours, or overnight, in an ice cube tray.

Serving Suggestion: Serve with whole-wheat toasted bread for breakfast.
Variation Tip: Add stevia as a natural sweetener.
Nutritional Information Per Serving:
Calories 492 | Protein 0g | Carbohydrate 7g | Dietary Fiber 1g | Sugar 0g | Fat 50g | Sodium 9mg

Apple and Peach Smoothie

Prep Time: 10 minutes
Servings: 4
Ingredients:
- 4 apples, peeled and chopped
- 4 cups mustard greens, chopped
- 4 peaches, peeled, cored, and chopped
- ½ teaspoon ground cinnamon
- 3 cups water
- ½ cup ice cubes

Preparation:
3. Add the ingredients to a high-speed blender and blend until smooth.
4. Pour into serving glasses and serve with a smile!

Serving Suggestion: Top with whipped cream before serving.
Variation Tip: You can also use coconut sugar to enhance the taste.
Nutritional Information per Serving:
Calories: 272|Fat: 2.3g |Sat Fat: 1.4g|Carbohydrates: 67g|Fiber: 13.9g|Sugar: 45.9g|Protein: 3.1g

Strawberry Spinach Smoothie

Prep Time: 10 minutes
Cook Time: 0 minutes
Serves: 2
Ingredients:
- 1 ripe banana, peeled and sliced
- 1 cup almond milk
- ½ cup strawberries, fresh
- 1 cup baby spinach, fresh
- 1 teaspoon spirulina powder
- 1 tablespoon hemp seeds
- 1 teaspoon vanilla extract
- 1 teaspoon Ceylon cinnamon powder
- 1 teaspoon baobab powder

Preparation:
1. Ready all the fruits and vegetables, then put them in a blender.
2. Toss in the rest of the smoothie ingredients.
3. Hit the pulse button to blend the smoothie until smooth.
4. Chill the smoothie for 2 hours in the refrigerator.
5. Serve chilled and fresh.

Serving Suggestion: Serve the smoothie with cranberry muffins.
Variation Tip: Add crushed pecans to the smoothie.
Nutritional Information per Serving:
Calories 217 | Fat 12g |Sodium 79mg | Carbs 28g | Fiber 1.1g | Sugar 18g | Protein 5g

Matcha Smoothie

Prep Time: 10 minutes
Cook Time: 0 minutes
Serves: 2
Ingredients:
- 2 cups ice cubes
- 1 cup almond milk
- ½ cup plain Greek yogurt
- 1 cup baby spinach
- 1 cup baby kale
- 1 banana, sliced
- ¼ cup almonds, sliced
- 1 tablespoon matcha tea powder
- 2 teaspoons erythritol

Preparation:
1. Ready all the fruits and vegetables, then put them in a blender.
2. Toss in the rest of the smoothie ingredients.
3. Hit the pulse button to blend the smoothie until smooth.
4. Chill the smoothie for 2 hours in the refrigerator.
5. Serve chilled and fresh.

Serving Suggestion: Serve the smoothie with pretzels.
Variation Tip: Add a few mint leaves to the smoothie.
Nutritional Information per Serving:
Calories 104 | Fat 4.2g |Sodium 62mg | Carbs 15g | Fiber 1g | Sugar 9g | Protein 5.6g

Muesli Breakfast Bars

Prep Time: 15 minutes
Cook Time: 25 minutes
Serves: 24
Ingredients
- 2½ cups old-fashioned rolled oats
- ½ cup soy flour
- ½ cup fat-free powdered milk
- ½ cup toasted wheat germ
- ½ cup sliced almonds or chopped pecans, toasted
- ½ cup chopped dried apples
- ½ cup raisins
- ½ tsp. salt
- 1 cup dark honey
- ½ cup natural unsalted peanut butter
- 1 tbsp. olive oil
- 2 tsp. vanilla extract

Preparation
1. Heat the oven to 325°F. Lightly coat a 9 x 13-inch baking pan with cooking spray.
2. Combine the oats, flour, dry milk, wheat germ, almonds, apples, raisins, and salt in a large bowl. Stir well to blend and set aside.
3. In a small saucepan, stir together the honey, peanut butter, and olive oil over medium-low heat until well-blended. Don't let the mixture boil. Stir in the vanilla.
4. Add the warm honey mixture to the dry ingredients and stir quickly until well-combined. The resulting mixture should be sticky but not wet.
5. Pat the mixture evenly into the prepared baking pan. Press firmly to remove any air pockets. Bake just until the edges begin to brown, about 25 minutes.
6. Let cool in the pan on a wire rack for 10 minutes, and then cut into 24 bars. When just cool enough to handle, remove the bars from the pan and place them on the rack to cool completely.
7. Store the bars in airtight containers in the refrigerator.

Serving Suggestion: Serve with tea.
Variation Tip: You can find fresh, sticky, moist dates to add to the mixture.
Nutritional Information Per Serving:
Calories 169 | Protein 5g | Carbohydrate 2g | Dietary fiber 2g | Sugar 11g | Fat 5g | Sodium 81mg

Banana Oatmeal Pancakes

Prep Time: 10 minutes
Cook Time: 10 minutes
Serves: 4
Ingredients
- ½ cup old-fashioned rolled oats
- 1 cup hot water or boiling water
- 2 tbsp. canola oil
- 2 tbsp. brown sugar
- ½ cup whole-wheat flour
- ½ cup all-purpose flour
- 1½ tsp. baking powder
- ¼ tsp. baking soda
- ¼ tsp. salt
- ¼ tsp. ground cinnamon
- ½ cup skim milk
- ¼ cup fat-free plain yogurt
- 1 mashed banana
- 1 egg

Preparation
1. In a large bowl, combine the oats and hot water. Let the mixture sit for 1 to 2 minutes until the oats are creamy and tender. Stir in the oil and sugar. Set aside to cool slightly.
2. Combine the flours, baking powder, baking soda, salt, and ground cinnamon in a medium bowl. Whisk to blend.
3. Add the milk, yogurt, and banana to the oats and stir until well-blended. Beat in the egg.
4. Add the flour mixture to the oat mixture and stir until just moistened.
5. Place a non-stick frying pan or skillet over medium heat. Once hot, spoon ¼ cup pancake batter into the pan. Cook for about 2 minutes or until the top surface of the pancake is covered with bubbles, and the edges are lightly browned. Flip the pancake and cook for another 2 to 3 minutes.
6. Repeat with the remaining pancake batter.

Serving Suggestion: Serve with tea.
Variation Tip: For a nuttier flavor, replace ¼ cup whole-wheat flour with ground flaxseeds or ground pumpkin seeds.
Nutritional Information Per Serving:
Calories 288 | Protein 9g | Carbohydrate 45g | Dietary fiber 3g | Sugars 12 g | Fat 9g | Sodium 453mg

Whole-Wheat Soda Bread

Prep Time: 20 minutes
Cook Time: 60 minutes
Serves: 16
Ingredients
- 2 cups whole-wheat flour
- 1 tsp. baking powder
- ¼ cup flaxseed meal (flaxseed flour)
- ½ tsp. baking soda
- ¼ cup millet meal (millet flour)
- 1 tsp. caraway seeds, crushed
- 2 tbsp. wheat gluten
- ¼ tsp. kosher salt
- 1¼ cup low-fat buttermilk or skim milk
- 2 egg whites

Preparation
1. Heat the oven to 350°F.
2. In a large bowl, sift together the dry ingredients.
3. In a separate bowl, combine the milk and egg whites. Mix well.
4. Add the milk and egg mixture to the dry ingredients. Mix until well-moistened.
5. Lightly grease the bottom of a 5 x 8-inch loaf pan. Place the dough in the pan. Using a sharp knife, make a slash in the dough lengthwise, about ¼ inch deep.
6. Bake for 50 to 60 minutes. To test for doneness, insert a skewer or knife into the center of the loaf. It should come out clean. Cool thoroughly on a rack before slicing.
Serving Suggestion: Serve with tea.
Variation Tip: You can top the bread with non-fat cream and nuts.
Nutritional Information Per Serving:
Calories 85 | Protein 5g | Carbohydrate 15g | Dietary fiber 2g | Sugar 0g | Fat 1g | Sodium 116mg

Carrot and Spice Quick Bread

Prep Time: 25 minutes
Cook Time: 45 minutes
Serves: 17
Ingredients
- ½ cup sifted all-purpose flour
- 1 cup whole-wheat flour
- 2 tsp. baking powder

- ½ tsp. baking soda
- ½ tsp. ground cinnamon
- ¼ tsp. ground ginger
- ⅓ cup trans-fat-free margarine, softened to room temperature
- ¼ cup, plus 2 tbsp., firmly packed brown sugar
- ⅓ cup skim milk
- 2 tbsp. unsweetened orange juice
- 2 egg whites, or egg substitute equivalent to 1 egg, beaten
- 1 tsp. vanilla extract
- 1 tsp. grated orange rind
- 1½ cups shredded carrots
- 2 tbsp. golden raisins
- 1 tbsp. finely chopped walnuts

Preparation
1. Heat the oven to 375°F. Grease a 2½ x 4½ x 8 ½-inch loaf pan with cooking spray.

2. In a small bowl, combine the first six dry ingredients. Set aside.
3. Using a mixer or stirring vigorously by hand, cream the margarine and sugar in a large bowl. Beat in the milk, orange juice, egg, vanilla, and orange rind. Stir in the carrots, raisins, and walnuts. Add the reserved dry ingredients. Mix well.
4. Spoon the batter into the loaf pan. Bake for 45 minutes, or until a wooden pick inserted in the center comes out clean. Cool in the pan for 10 minutes. Remove from the pan and let cool completely on a wire rack.
Serving Suggestion: Serve with tea.
Variation Tip: You can add chopped nuts to the mixture before cooking.
Nutritional Information Per Serving:
Calories 110 | Protein 2g | Carbohydrate 15g | Dietary fiber 1g | Sugar 6g | Fat 5g | Sodium 82mg

Spiced Carrot and Raisin Tea Bread

Prep Time: 15 minutes
Cook Time: 60 minutes
Serves: 18
Ingredients
- 1½ cup whole-wheat pastry flour
- ¼ cup flaxseed flour
- ½ tsp. baking soda
- 1½ tsp. baking powder
- ½ tsp. salt
- 1 tbsp. cinnamon
- ½ tsp. nutmeg
- ¼ tsp. cloves

- ¼ tsp. ground cayenne pepper
- 2 eggs
- ½ cup brown sugar
- ¼ cup honey
- ½ cup unsweetened applesauce
- ¼ cup olive oil
- ¾ tsp. almond extract
- 1 tbsp. grated lemon zest
- 2 cups shredded carrots (about 4 carrots in total)
- ²/₃ cup raisins

Preparation
1. Heat the oven to 375°F.
2. Sift the wheat and flax flours, baking soda, baking powder, salt, and spices into a large bowl. Whisk until combined.
3. Mix the eggs, brown sugar, honey, applesauce, olive oil, and almond extract in a separate bowl. Stir in the lemon zest, carrots, and raisins.
4. Add the wet ingredients to the dry ingredients and stir until just combined, being careful not to over mix.
5. Pour the batter into a lightly greased 9 x 5-inch loaf pan and bake for 45 to 60 minutes until a tester inserted into the center comes out clean.

Serving Suggestion: Cool and cut into ½-inch slices and serve.
Variation Tip: You can add flaxseed flour and spices, including cayenne pepper, to give this tea bread a rich flavor.
Nutritional Information Per Serving:
Calories 144 | Protein 2g | Carbohydrate 25g | Dietary fiber 3g | Sugar 10g | Fat 4g | Sodium 140mg

Whole-Grain Pancakes

Prep Time: 15 minutes
Cook Time: 15 minutes
Serves: 9
Ingredients
- 1 cup whole-wheat flour
- ¼ cup millet flour
- ½ cup barley flour
- 2 tbsp. flaxseed flour
- ¼ cup rolled oats
- 1½ tbsp. baking powder
- 3 tbsp. honey
- 1 tbsp. oil
- 2¼ cups soy milk
- 3 large egg whites, beaten

Preparation

1. In a large bowl, mix the dry ingredients together.
2. Mix the wet ingredients (honey, oil, soy milk, and beaten egg whites) in a separate bowl.
3. Add the egg mixture to the dry ingredients. Stir until just combined. Let the batter rest for 30 minutes in the refrigerator.
4. Place a baking sheet in the oven and heat to 225°F.
5. Place a frying pan on medium heat. Spoon or ladle about ¼ cup of batter into the pan to make one pancake. Cook until small bubbles form and the edges begin to look dry. Flip and cook until brown on the second side.
6. Transfer the pancake to the baking sheet to keep warm. Repeat with the remaining batter.

Serving Suggestion: Top the pancakes with fresh fruit.
Variation Tip: You can serve with low-fat cream or a honey topping.
Nutritional Information Per Serving:
Calories 180 | Protein 6g | Carbohydrate 30g | Dietary fiber 4g | Sugar 6g | Fat 4g | Sodium 168mg

Cinnamon Rolls

Prep Time: 1 hour 40 minutes
Cook Time: 25 minutes
Serves: 32
Ingredients
- 1 cup skim milk
- ¼ cup canola oil
- ⅓ cup sugar
- ¼ tsp. salt
- 2 packets dry yeast (about 0.75 oz. per packet)
- ¼ cup warm water
- 1 egg
- 2 egg whites
- 3 cups all-purpose (plain) flour
- 2½ cups whole-wheat (whole-meal) flour
- Cooking spray
- 2 tbsp. ground cinnamon
- ¾ cup brown sugar
- ¼ cup raisins
- ½ cup frozen unsweetened apple juice concentrate, thawed

Preparation
1. In a small saucepan, heat the milk until just below the boiling point. Don't boil.
2. Stir in the canola oil, sugar, and salt. Remove the milk mixture from the heat and cool until lukewarm.
3. In a small bowl, combine the yeast and water. Stir and set aside for 5 minutes.
4. In a large bowl, beat the egg and egg whites using an electric mixer. Add in the yeast and milk mixture.
5. Using a wooden spoon, mix in the flours, 1 cup at a time, until a soft dough forms. (If you have a countertop mixer, use a dough hook and follow the manufacturer's directions.)

6. Turn the dough out onto a generously floured work surface. With floured hands, knead gently until the dough is smooth and elastic, about 5 minutes.

7. Return the dough to the bowl and cover with plastic wrap. Let rise in a warm place until double in size, about 1½ hours.

8. Divide the dough in half and form it into 2 balls. Cover with plastic and let it sit for 10 more minutes.

9. In a small bowl, combine the cinnamon, brown sugar, and raisins.

10. Spray an 11 x 14-inch pan with cooking spray.

11. Using a rolling pin, roll each ball of dough into a 16 x 8-inch rectangle. Spray the dough with cooking/baking spray.

12. Sprinkle each rectangle with half of the cinnamon mixture. Starting at the long side, roll up each rectangle. Slice each roll into 16 pieces and place them on the prepared pan. Let them rise until double in size, about 1½ hours.

13. To make the glaze, heat the apple juice over medium heat. Cook until the liquid is syrupy, about 5 to 7 minutes. Set aside.

14. Heat the oven to 350°F. Brush each roll with the glaze. Bake until golden brown (about 15 minutes).

15. If you want to freeze the rolls for later, only bake them until the dough rises a bit more but hasn't browned. Cool the partially baked rolls in the pan. Wrap the rolls tightly in 2 layers of plastic wrap and freeze. When you want to use them, thaw them in the refrigerator. Then bake at 350°F for 8-10 minutes.

Serving Suggestion: Serve the rolls warm.

Variation Tip: You can top the rolls with low-fat cream or honey if desired.

Nutritional Information Per Serving:
Calories 130 | Protein 3g | Carbohydrate 25g | Dietary fiber 2g | Sugar 8g | Fat 2g | Sodium 30mg

Cinnamon French Toast

Prep Time: 5 minutes
Cook Time: 5 minutes
Serves: 2
Ingredients
- 4 egg whites
- 1 tsp. vanilla
- $1/8$ tsp. ground nutmeg
- 4 slices cinnamon bread
- ¼ tsp. ground cinnamon

- ¼ cup maple syrup

Preparation

1. In a small bowl, combine the egg whites, vanilla, and nutmeg. Whisk to mix evenly.

2. Dip the bread into the egg mixture, coating both sides.

3. Place a non-stick frying pan or skillet over medium heat. When a drop of water sizzles as it hits the pan, add the bread. Sprinkle with cinnamon. Cook until both sides are golden brown, about 4 to 5 minutes on each side.

4. Place two slices of French toast on warmed individual plates. Add 1 tbsp. of maple syrup to each.

Serving Suggestion: Serve with tea.

Variation Tip: You can add some sweetener to the egg mixture.

Nutritional Information Per Serving:
Calories 299 | Protein 11g | Carbohydrate 57g | Dietary fiber 1g | Sugar 17g | Fat 3g | Sodium 334mg

Southwestern Cornmeal Muffins

Prep Time: 10 minutes
Cook Time: 20 minutes
Serves: 12
Ingredients
- 1 cup all-purpose flour
- ¼ cup sugar
- 2 tsp. baking powder
- 1 cup fat-free milk
- 4 tbsp. (or ¼ cup) vegetable oil
- ½ cup egg substitute
- 1¼ cups stone-ground cornmeal
- 1 cup fresh or cream-style corn
- ½ green bell pepper, chopped

Preparation

1. Heat the oven to 400°F. Line a muffin pan with paper or foil liners.

2. In a large bowl, add the flour, sugar, and baking powder. Stir to mix evenly.

3. Combine the milk, oil, egg substitute, cornmeal, corn, and green pepper in a separate bowl. Add to the flour mixture and blend just until moistened but still slightly lumpy.

4. Divide the mixture among the 12 muffin liners. Bake for 20 minutes or until the muffins are light brown.

Serving Suggestion: Serve with tea.

Variation Tip: Add nuts if you want.

Nutritional Information Per Serving:
Calories 168 | Protein 4g | Carbohydrate 26g | Dietary fiber 1.5g | Sugar 4g | Fat 5g | Sodium 156 mg

Strawberry Breakfast Sandwich

Prep Time: 10 minutes
Cook Time: 0 minutes
Serves: 4
Ingredients:
• 1 tablespoon honey
• 8 ounces low-fat cream cheese, softened
• 1 teaspoon grated lemon zest
• 4 English muffins, split and toasted
• 2 cups (about 10 ounces) sliced strawberries
Preparation:
1. Blend the cheese, zest, and cheese in a food processor.
2. Spread the cheese mixture over one-half of the muffin.
3. Top it with strawberries.
4. Place the other muffin slice on top.
Serving Suggestion: Serve the meal with a glass of kiwi smoothie.
Variation Tip: Sprinkle roasted nuts over the berries.
Nutritional Information per Serving:
Calories 284 | Fat 7.9g |Sodium 54mg | Carbs 37g | Fiber 3.6g | Sugar 6g | Protein 11g

Popovers

Prep Time: 15 minutes
Cook Time: 35 minutes
Serves: 6
Ingredients
• 1 cup skim milk
• 1 cup all-purpose (plain) flour
• ¼ tsp. salt
• 4 egg whites
Preparation
1. Heat the oven to 425°F.
2. Generously coat six large metal or glass muffin molds with cooking spray. Heat the muffin molds in the oven for 2 minutes.
3. In a large bowl, add the milk, flour, salt, and egg whites. Using an electric mixer, beat until smooth.

4. Fill the heated muffin molds ⅔ full. Bake in the top part of the oven until golden brown and puffy, about 30 minutes.
Serving Suggestion: Serve immediately with tea.
Variation Tip: Add some sweetener to the mixture if you want.
Nutritional Information Per Serving:
Calories 96 | Protein 6g | Carbohydrate 18g | Dietary fiber 0.5g | Sugar 2g | Fat 0.1g | Sodium 156mg

Turkey and Mushroom Strata

Prep Time: 10 minutes
Cook Time: 63 minutes
Serves: 6
Ingredients:
• 8 ounces wheat ciabatta bread, cubed
• 12 ounces turkey sausage
• 2 cups fat-free milk
• 1½ cups reduced-fat cheese, shredded
• 12 ounces egg substitute
• ½ cup chopped green onion
• 1 cup sliced mushrooms
• ½ teaspoon paprika
• Fresh ground pepper to taste
• 2 tablespoons grated parmesan cheese
Preparation:
1. Preheat your oven to 400°F.
2. Add the bread pieces to a baking sheet in a single layer.
3. Bake in the oven for 8 minutes.
4. Sauté the sausage in a pan for 7 minutes, constantly stirring.
5. Mix the milk with the eggs, parmesan, cheese, paprika, pepper, and egg substitute.
6. Stir in the baked bread cubes, scallions, sausages, and mushrooms.
7. Transfer the mixture to a 13-inch x 9-inch baking dish.
8. Cover and refrigerate the dish for 8 hours.
9. Preheat the oven to 350°F.
10. Bake the casserole for 50 minutes.
11. Slice and serve.
Serving Suggestion: Serve the meal with a glass of avocado smoothie.
Variation Tip: Sprinkle cheese over the strata before serving.
Nutritional Information per Serving:
Calories 248 | Fat 12g |Sodium 121mg | Carbs 26g | Fiber 4g | Sugar 8g | Protein 7g

Overnight Oatmeal

Prep Time: 15 minutes
Cook Time: 0 minutes
Serves: 8
Ingredients:
- 4 cups fat-free milk
- 4 cups water
- 2 cups steel-cut oats
- ⅓ cup dried cherries
- ⅓ cup raisins
- ⅓ cup dried apricots, chopped
- 1 teaspoon molasses
- 1 teaspoon cinnamon

Preparation:
1. Add the oats, milk, water, and the rest of the ingredients to a bowl.
2. Divide into four mason jars, cover the jars and refrigerate overnight.
3. Serve.

Serving Suggestion: Serve the meal with a glass of mint smoothie.
Variation Tip: Replace blueberries with strawberries for change of flavor.
Nutritional Information per Serving:
Calories 117 | Fat 13g |Sodium 34mg | Carbs 31g | Fiber 1g | Sugar 10g | Protein 11g

Fruit Grain Salad

Prep Time: 10 minutes
Cook Time: 10 minutes
Serves: 4
Ingredients:
- 3 cups water
- ¼ teaspoon salt
- ¾ cup quick-cooking brown rice
- ¾ cup bulgur
- 1 Granny Smith apple
- 1 Red Delicious apple
- 1 orange
- 1 cup raisins
- 8 ounces low-fat vanilla yogurt

Preparation:
1. Add the water to a large pot and boil it over high heat.
2. Stir in the bulgur and rice and cook on low heat for 10 minutes.
3. Spread the cooked grains on a baking sheet and refrigerate overnight.
4. Toss the mixed grains with all the fruits in a bowl.
5. Stir in the yogurt and serve.

Serving Suggestion: Serve the meal with a glass of apple smoothie.
Variation Tip: Sprinkle shaved coconut over the breakfast salad.
Nutritional Information per Serving:
Calories 212 | Fat 3.9g |Sodium 95mg | Carbs 14.3g | Fiber 5.2g | Sugar3.2g | Protein 5.3g

Baked Oatmeal

Prep Time: 15 minutes
Cook Time: 30 minutes
Serves: 8
Ingredients
- 1 tbsp. canola oil
- ½ cup unsweetened applesauce
- ⅓ cup brown sugar
- Egg substitute equivalent to 2 eggs, or 4 egg whites
- 3 cups uncooked rolled oats
- 2 tsp. baking powder
- 1 tsp. cinnamon
- 1 cup skim milk

Preparation
1. Preheat the oven to 350°F.
2. In a good-sized bowl, stir together the oil, applesauce, sugar, and eggs.
3. Add the dry ingredients and milk. Mix well.
4. Spray a 9 x 13-inch baking pan generously with cooking spray. Spoon the oatmeal mixture into the pan. Bake uncovered for 30 minutes.

Serving Suggestion: Serve hot with sliced bananas, strawberries, blueberries, and a drizzle of honey.
Variation Tip: You can mix this in the evening and refrigerate it overnight. Just pop it in the oven first thing when you get up.
Nutritional Information Per Serving:
Calories 196 | Protein 7g | Carbohydrate 33g | Dietary fiber 3g | Sugar 8.5g | Fat 4g | Sodium 105mg

Spinach Mushroom Scramble

Prep Time: 15 minutes
Cook Time: 10 minutes
Serves: 4
Ingredients:
• Cooking spray
• ½ cup fresh mushrooms, sliced
• 1 cup fresh spinach, chopped
• 1 whole egg
• 2 egg whites
• 2 tablespoons feta cheese
• Pepper to taste
Preparation:
1. Sauté the mushrooms with the spinach in a pan over medium heat for 3 minutes.
2. Whisk the egg with the egg whites and feta cheese.
3. Pour the mixture into the skillet.
4. Cook for 2 to 3 minutes, then scramble.
5. Cook for another 1 to 2 minutes.
6. Serve warm.
Serving Suggestion: Serve the meal with a glass of matcha smoothie.
Variation Tip: Add chopped carrots and onion to the scramble.
Nutritional Information per Serving:
Calories 234 | Fat 4.7g |Sodium 41mg | Carbs 18g | Fiber 7g | Sugar 3.3g | Protein 6g

Omelet Waffles

Prep Time: 10 minutes
Cook Time: 5 minutes
Serves: 2
Ingredients:

• 4 eggs
• A pinch of black pepper
• 2 tablespoons ham, chopped
• ¼ cup low-fat cheddar, shredded
• 2 tablespoons parsley, chopped
• Cooking spray
Preparation:
1. Combine the eggs with pepper, ham, cheese and parsley in a bowl and whisk effectively.
2. Grease your waffle iron with cooking spray, add the egg mix, cook for 4-5 minutes.
3. Divide the waffles between plates and serve them for breakfast.
4. Enjoy!
Serving Suggestion: Garnish with chives.
Variation Tip: Substitute Cheddar with Parmesan cheese.
Nutritional Information per Serving:
Calories 200 | Fat 7g | Sodium 350mg | Carbs 29g | Fiber 3g | Sugar 0g | Protein 3g

Easy Salmon Cakes

Prep Time: 45 minutes
Cook Time: 20 minutes
Serves: 4
Ingredients
• 3 tsp. extra-virgin olive oil, divided
• 1 small onion, finely chopped
• 1 stalk celery, finely diced
• 2 tbsp. chopped fresh parsley
• 15 oz. canned salmon, drained, or 1½ cups cooked salmon
• 1 large egg, lightly beaten
• 1½ tsp. Dijon mustard
• 1¾ cups fresh whole-wheat breadcrumbs
• ½ tsp. freshly ground pepper
• 1 lemon, cut into wedges
Preparation
1. Preheat the oven to 450°F. Coat a baking sheet with cooking spray.
2. Heat 1½ tsp. of the oil in a large non-stick skillet over medium-high heat. Add the onion and celery. Cook, stirring, until softened, for about 3 minutes. Stir in the parsley and remove from the heat.
3. Place the salmon in a medium bowl. Flake it apart with a fork. Remove any bones and skin.
4. Add the egg and mustard. Mix well.
5. Add the onion mixture, breadcrumbs, and pepper. Mix well.

6. Shape the mixture into eight patties, about 2½ inches wide.

7. Heat the remaining oil in the pan over medium heat. Add four patties and cook until the undersides are golden, 2 to 3 minutes. Using a wide spatula, turn them over onto the prepared baking sheet. Repeat with the remaining patties.

8. Bake the salmon cakes until golden on top and heated through (about 15 to 20 minutes).

Serving Suggestion: Serve salmon cakes with the lemon wedges and a low-fat yogurt dip.

Variation Tip: Add spices of your choice to the fish mixture before cooking.

Nutritional Information Per Serving:
Calories 350 | Protein 34.4g | Carbohydrates 25.8g | Dietary fiber 5.7g | Sugars 5.5g | Fat 13.7g | Sodium 761.4mg

Chickpea Polenta with Olives

Prep Time: 15 minutes
Cook Time: 21 minutes
Serves: 6
Ingredients:
Polenta:
• 1¾ cups chickpea flour
• 2 cups plain soy milk
• 1 cup low-sodium chicken stock
• ½ tablespoon olive oil
• 3 garlic cloves, chopped
• 1 tablespoon fresh thyme, chopped
• 1 teaspoon dry mustard
• ¼ teaspoon black pepper
• 3 egg whites
Topping:
• ½ tablespoon olive oil
• ½ yellow onion, minced
• ¼ cup pitted Kalamata olives, chopped
• ¼ cup dry-packed sun-dried tomatoes, chopped
• 2 tablespoons grated parmesan cheese
• 2 tablespoons flat-leaf parsley, chopped
Preparation:
1. Blend the flour with the soy milk, olive oil, thyme, garlic, stock, pepper, and mustard in a food processor.
2. Let this batter refrigerate for 1 hour.
3. Preheat the oven to 425°F. Grease a 9-inch x 13-inch baking pan with cooking oil.
4. Pour the batter into the pan and bake for 15 minutes, then allow it to cool.
5. Meanwhile, preheat the broiler and set the racks about 4 inches from the heat source.
6. Heat a skillet with olive oil and sauté the onion for 6 minutes.
7. Stir in the tomatoes and olives. Stir and cook for 1 minute.

8. Spoon this mixture over the baked polenta and sprinkle the cheese on top.
9. Broil the polenta for 1 minute, then allow it cool for 10 minutes.
10. Cut the polenta into 16 wedges and garnish with parsley.
11. Serve.

Serving Suggestion: Serve the polenta with a smoothie of your choice.

Variation Tip: Add chopped herbs on top.

Nutritional Information per Serving:
Calories 157 | Fat 3.9g |Sodium 135mg | Carbs 24g | Fiber 1g | Sugar 0g | Protein 4.5g

Cranberry Orange Muffins

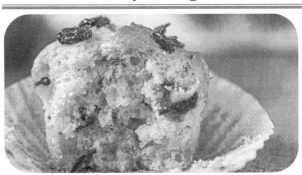

Prep Time: 10 minutes
Cook Time: 22 minutes
Serves: 6
Ingredients:
• 8 ounces Greek yogurt
• 2 eggs
• ¼ cup canola oil
• ½ cup granulated sugar
• ¼ cup brown sugar
• 2 tablespoons orange juice
• 2 tablespoons orange zest
• 2 teaspoons vanilla
• ¼ flaxseed meal
• 1 teaspoon baking powder
• 1 teaspoon baking soda
• 1¾ cups all-purpose flour
• ½ teaspoon cinnamon
• $\frac{1}{8}$ teaspoon salt
• 1½ cups frozen cranberries
Preparation:
1. Grease a muffin tin with cooking spray. Preheat the oven to 350°F.
2. Whisk the eggs with the sugars, oil, yogurt, orange zest, vanilla, and orange juice in a bowl.
3. Combine the flaxseed with the baking powder, cinnamon, salt, flour, and baking soda in another bowl.
4. Mix both the dry and wet mixtures in a large bowl at low speed until well combined.
5. Fold in the cranberries after 2 minutes of mixing.
6. Put the batter into the muffin cups.
7. Bake them for 22 minutes until golden brown.
8. Serve with desired garnish.

Serving Suggestion: Serve the meal with a glass of apple smoothie.

Variation Tip: Add mini chocolate chips to the batter.

Nutritional Information per Serving:
Calories 240 | Fat 5g |Sodium 44mg | Carbs 26g | Fiber 1g | Sugar 1g | Protein 2g

Buckwheat Crepes

Prep Time: 10 minutes
Cook Time: 15 minutes
Serves: 6
Ingredients:
- 1 cup buckwheat flour
- ⅓ cup whole grain flour
- 1 egg, beaten
- 1 cup skim milk
- 1 teaspoon olive oil
- ½ teaspoon ground cinnamon

Preparation:
1. In the mixing bowl, mix up all ingredients and whisk until you get a smooth batter.
2. Heat the non-stick skillet on high heat for 3 minutes.
3. Using a ladle, pour the small amount of batter into the skillet and flatten it in the shape of a crepe.
4. Cook it for 1 minute and flip on another side. Cook it for 30 seconds more.
5. Repeat the same steps with the remaining batter.

Serving Suggestion: Serve with vanilla yogurt, garnished with your favorite berries.
Variation Tip: Swap buckwheat with whole wheat flour.
Nutritional Information per Serving:
Calories 122 | Fat 2.2g | Sodium 34 mg | Carbs 211.g | Fiber 2g | Sugar 5g | Protein 5.7g

Oatmeal Banana Pancakes with Walnuts

Prep Time: 10 minutes
Cook Time: 5 minutes
Serves: 8 pancakes
Ingredients:
- 1 finely diced firm banana
- 1 cup whole wheat pancake mix
- ⅛ cup chopped walnuts
- ¼ cup old-fashioned oats

Preparation:
1. Make the pancake mix according to the directions on the package.
2. Add walnuts, oats and chopped bananas.
3. Coat a griddle with cooking spray.
4. Add about ¼ cup of the pancake batter onto the griddle when hot.
5. Turn pancake over when bubbles form on top. Cook until golden brown.
6. Serve immediately.

Serving Suggestion: Garnish with banana slices.
Variation Tip: Feel free to substitute walnuts with your favorite nuts.
Nutritional Information per Serving:
Calories 155 | Fat 4g | Sodium 16mg | Carbs 28g | Fiber 7g | Sugar 2.2g | Protein 7g

Oats, Buckwheat and Seeds Granola

Prep Time: 10 minutes
Cook Time: 40 minutes
Serves: 6
Ingredients:
- 1 cup oats
- ½ cup buckwheat
- ½ cup sunflower seeds
- ½ cup pumpkin seeds
- ¾ cup dates, pitted
- ¼ cup olive oil
- 1½ tablespoons cocoa powder
- ½ cup apple puree

Preparation:
1. Preheat the baking oven to 350° F.
2. Meanwhile, add seeds, buckwheat and oats in a bowl. Mix well.
3. Now, heat oil in a pan and cook dates and apple puree in it for about four to five minutes.
4. Add the date mixture in the oat mixture and stir properly.
5. Transfer the mixture in the baking sheet and bake for about 35 minutes. Stirring occasionally.
6. Take out and set aside to cool.
7. Stir in cocoa powder and serve.

Serving Suggestions: Sprinkle chocolate chips on the top before serving.
Variation Tip: Cocoa powder can be omitted.
Nutritional Information per Serving:
Calories: 335 | Fat: 18.3g | Sat Fat: 2.9g | Carbohydrates: 41.6g | Fiber: 6.6g | Sugar: 17.7g | Protein: 8.9g

Granola Parfait

Prep Time: 10 minutes
Cook Time: 0 minutes
Serves: 2
Ingredients:
• ½ cup low-fat yogurt
• 4 tablespoons granolas
Preparation:
1. Put ½ tablespoon of granola in every glass.
2. Then add 2 tablespoons of low-fat yogurt.
3. Repeat the steps till you use all ingredients.
4. Store the parfait in the fridge for up to 2 hours.
Serving Suggestion: Top with berries of your choice.
Variation Tip: Feel free to use vanilla Greek yogurt.
Nutritional Information per Serving:
Calories 79 | Fat 8.1 g | Sodium 51 mg | Carbs 20.6 g | Fiber 2.8 g | Sugar 10.4 g| Protein 8 g

Breakfast Hash

Prep Time: 10 minutes
Cook Time: 25 minutes
Serves: 4
Ingredients:
• Non-stick cooking spray
• 2 large sweet potatoes, peeled and cut into ½-inch cubes
• 1 scallion, finely chopped
• ¼ teaspoon salt
• ½ teaspoon freshly ground black pepper
• 8 ounces extra-lean ground beef (96% or leaner)
• 1 medium onion, sliced
• 2 garlic cloves, minced
• 1 red bell pepper, diced
• ¼ teaspoon ground cumin
• ¼ teaspoon paprika
• 2 cups coarsely chopped kale leaves
• ¾ cup shredded reduced-fat Cheddar cheese
• 4 large eggs
Preparation:

1. Coat a large skillet with cooking spray and heat over medium heat. Add sweet potatoes, scallion, salt and pepper.
2. Sauté for 10 minutes, stirring
3. Add the beef, onion, garlic, bell pepper, cumin and paprika. Sauté, frequently stirring, for about 4 minutes, or until the meat browns.
4. Add the kale skillet and stir until wilted. Sprinkle with the Cheddar cheese.
5. Make four wells in the mixture and put an egg into each well.
Cover and the eggs cook until the white is fully cooked and the yolk is to your preference.
Serving Suggestion: Garnish with parsley
Variation Tip: Feel free to swap red bell peppers with yellow bell peppers
Nutritional Information per Serving:
Calories 323 | Fat 1 5g | Sodium 587 mg | Carbs 23 g | Fiber4 g | Sugar 14g | Protein 25 g

Quiche Muffins

Prep Time: 10 minutes
Cook Time: 40 minutes
Serves: 6
Ingredients:
• 1 cup green onion, chopped
• ¾ cup low-fat cheese, shredded
• 1 cup broccoli, chopped
• 1 cup tomatoes, diced
• 2 cups non-fat or 1% milk
• 4 eggs
• 1 cup baking mix
• 1 teaspoon Italian seasoning
• ½ teaspoon salt
• ½ teaspoon black pepper
Preparation:
1. Preheat the oven to 375°F. Grease a 12-muffin tray with oil.
2. Add the cheese, onions, tomatoes, and broccoli into each muffin cup.
3. Beat all the remaining ingredients in a bowl.
4. Divide this mixture into each muffin cup.
5. Bake for 40 minutes in the oven.
6. Allow it to cool.
Serving Suggestion: Serve the meal with a glass of spinach smoothie.
Variation Tip: Sprinkle cheese over the quiches.
Nutritional Information per Serving:
Calories 217 | Fat 15g |Sodium 132mg | Carbs 29g | Fiber 3.9g | Sugar 3g |Protein 8.9g

Baked Eggs in Avocado

Prep Time: 10 minutes
Cook Time: 15 minutes
Serves: 2
Ingredients:
• 2 avocados
• Juice of 2 limes
• black pepper to taste
• 4 eggs
• 2 (8-inch) whole-wheat or corn tortillas, warmed
• Optional for serving: halved cherry tomatoes and chopped cilantro
Preparation:
1. Adjust the oven rack to the middle position and preheat the oven to 450° F. Scrape out the center of halved avocado using a spoon of about 1½ tablespoons.
2. Press lime juice over the avocados and season with black pepper to taste and then place it on a baking sheet. Crack two eggs into each avocado.
3. Bake within 10 to 15 minutes. Remove from oven and garnish with optional cilantro and cherry tomatoes.
Serving Suggestion: Serve with warm tortillas.
Variation Tip: Add in a teaspoon of smoked paprika for a vibrant taste.
Nutritional Information per Serving:
Calories 534 | Fat 39 g | Sodium 462 mg | Carbs 30 g | Fiber 20 g | Sugar 3 g | Protein 23 g

Veggie Toasts

Prep Time: 10 minutes
Cook Time: 15 minutes
Serves: 2
Ingredients:
• 1 red bell pepper
• 1 cup Cremini mushrooms; sliced
• 4 bread slices
• 2 tablespoons butter; soft
• 1 yellow squash; chopped.

• 2 green onions; sliced
• 1 tablespoon olive oil
• ½ cup Goat cheese, crumbled
Preparation:
1. Cut red bell pepper into thin strips. Mix red bell pepper with mushrooms, squash, green onions and oil, toss in a bowl.
2. Move to your air fryer and cook them at a temperature of 350° F for about 10 minutes.
3. Shake the fryer once and transfer them into a bowl.
4. Spread butter on bread slices, then introduce them to your air fryer and cook them at a temperature of 350° F. Cook for about 5 minutes.
5. Cut the veggie mix on each bread slice.
Serving Suggestion: Use crumbled cheese as toppings.
Variation Tip: Feel free to use yellow bell peppers.
Nutritional Information per Serving:
Calories 112 | Fat 1.58g | Sodium 219mg | Carbs 21g | Fiber 1g | Sugar 2g | Protein 3g

Mushroom Frittata

Prep Time: 10 minutes
Cook Time: 30 minutes
Serves: 2
Ingredients:
• 1 tablespoon unsalted butter
• 4 shallots, finely chopped
• ½-pound mushrooms
• 2 tablespoon fresh parsley, finely chopped
• 1 teaspoon dried thyme
• 3 eggs
• black pepper to taste
• 5 large egg whites
• 1 tablespoon milk or fat-free half-and-half
• ¼ cup fresh-grated Parmesan cheese
Preparation:
1. Preheat oven to 350° F.
2. Warm and melt butter in a large, oven-safe skillet. Stir in shallots and sauté until golden brown.
3. Add parsley, thyme, mushrooms and black pepper.
4. In another bowl, then whisk eggs and egg whites together with Parmesan cheese and milk.
5. Add the egg mixture to the skillet. When the edges begin to set, place the entire skillet in the oven.
6. Bake until frittata is fully cooked, about 15 minutes.
7. Cut into four wedges and serve.
Serving Suggestion: Garnish with parsley.
Variation Tip: Feel free to use any mushroom of your liking.
Nutritional Information per Serving:
Calories 132 | Fat 7g | Sodium 359mg | Carbs 6g | Fiber 0g | Sugar 0.1g | Protein 10g

Green Smoothie Bowl

Prep Time: 15 minutes
Serves: 4

Ingredients:
- 1 cup avocado, peeled, pitted and chopped
- 2 teaspoons fresh lime zest
- 1½ cups unsweetened coconut milk
- 2 cups fresh baby spinach
- 4 tablespoons fresh lime juice
- 1 teaspoon organic vanilla extract
- 8 drops liquid stevia

Preparation:
1. Add avocado, lime zest, unsweetened coconut milk, baby spinach, lime juice, vanilla extract and liquid stevia in a blender.
2. Blend until a smooth mixture is formed and transfer in four serving bowls.
3. Serve and enjoy!

Serving Suggestions: Top with fruits before serving.
Variation Tip: Stevia can be omitted.
Nutritional Information per Serving:
Calories: 851 | Fat: 85.9g | Sat Fat: 71.3g | Carbohydrates: 26g | Fiber: 10.4g | Sugar: 12.2g | Protein: 8.9g

Yogurt and Granola Bowl

Prep Time: 5 minutes
Serves: 2
Ingredients:
- 1 cup fat-free plain Greek yogurt
- ¼ cup oat granola
- ¼ cup fresh blueberries
- ½ banana, peeled and sliced
- 1 tablespoon walnut, chopped

Preparation:
1. Add blueberries, granola and yogurt in a bowl and stir well.
2. Divide the mixture in two bowls and top with banana slices and walnuts.
3. Serve and enjoy!

Serving Suggestions: Top with chopped almonds before serving.
Variation Tip: You can add honey for sweeter taste.
Nutritional Information per Serving:
Calories: 185 | Fat: 4.4g | Sat Fat: 1.2g | Carbohydrates: 24g | Fiber: 2.4g | Sugar: 13.2g | Protein: 14.7g

Apple Porridge

Prep Time: 5 minutes
Cook Time: 4 minutes
Serves: 2
Ingredients:
- 1 cup unsweetened almond milk
- ¼ teaspoon organic vanilla extract
- 2 tablespoons unsalted walnuts, chopped and divided
- 1½ tablespoons sunflower seeds
- ¼ apple, cored and sliced

Preparation:
1. Add milk, vanilla extract, sunflower seeds, apple and one tablespoon walnuts in a large pan. Mix well.
2. Cook for about four minutes on medium-low heat and take out.
3. Serve and enjoy!

Serving Suggestions: Top with apple slices before serving.
Variation Tip: Cinnamon can be added to enhance taste.
Nutritional Information per Serving:
Calories: 272 | Fat: 23.9g | Sat Fat: 2g | Carbohydrates: 10.5g | Fiber: 3.9g | Sugar: 3.2g | Protein: 6.2g

Banana Oatmeal

Prep Time: 10 minutes
Cook Time: 20 minutes
Serves: 2
Ingredients:
• 2 cups water
• ½ cup steel cut oats
• ½ banana, mashed
• ½ cup strawberries, hulled and sliced
Preparation: Add water and oats in a pan and simmer them over medium-high heat for 20 minutes.
1. Take out and set aside to cool.
2. Now, add in mashed banana and stir properly.
3. Top with strawberries and serve.
Serving Suggestions: Top with chopped pecans before serving.
Variation Tip: Cinnamon can be added to enhance taste.
Nutritional Information per Serving:
Calories: 115 | Fat: 1.5g | Sat Fat: 0.3g | Carbohydrates: 23.4g | Fiber: 3.6g | Sugar: 5.6g | Protein: 3.3g

Sweet Potato and Black Bean Hash

Prep Time: 10 minutes
Cook Time: 10 minutes
Serves: 3
Ingredients:
• 1 tablespoon extra-virgin olive oil
• 1 cup diced peeled sweet potato
• 1 (15 ounces, 425 g) can black beans, rinsed and drained
• 1 cup cauliflower rice
• 4 cherry tomatoes, halved
• 2 cups baby kale, stems removed, finely chopped
• 1 teaspoon sweet paprika
• Pinch of freshly ground black pepper
• 1-ounce unsalted roasted pumpkin seeds
• ¼ cup chopped fresh cilantro
Preparation:
1. Heat the oil over medium-high heat in a medium saucepan for about 30 seconds until shimmering.
2. Put in the sweet potato and cook about 5 minutes, frequently stirring until softened and lightly browned.
3. Stir in the beans, paprika, tomatoes, riced cauliflower, kale and black pepper. Continue cooking over medium heat for about 5 minutes until the beans are heated, and the kale has wilted.
4. Remove from the heat and divide onto three plates.
Serving Suggestion: Top with the pumpkin seeds and cilantro.
Variation Tip: Substitute the extra virgin olive oil with coconut oil.
Nutritional Information per Serving:
Calories 298| Fat 10 g | Sodium 45 mg | Carbs 42 g | Fiber 12 g | Sugar 5 g | Protein 14 g

Banana Cream Chia Pudding

Prep Time: 5 minutes
Cook Time: 0 minutes
Serves: 1
Ingredients:
• ¼ cup chia seeds
• ½ cup full-fat coconut milk
• ½ cup almond milk
• 1 tablespoon agave syrup
• 1 teaspoon cinnamon
• 1 banana, mashed
Preparation:
1. Blend the banana mash with the milk, agave, and cinnamon in a blender.
2. Stir in the chia seeds and leave to chill in the refrigerator for 15 minutes.
3. Serve chilled.
Serving Suggestion: Serve the pudding in a glass with banana slices on top.
Variation Tip: Add shredded coconut to the pudding.
Nutritional Information per Serving:
Calories 180 | Fat 19g |Sodium 18mg | Carbs 19g | Fiber 5g | Sugar 3g | Protein 6g

Wheat Berries and Fruits Bowl

Prep Time: 10 minutes
Cook Time: 38 minutes
Serves: 2
Ingredients:
- ¾ cup water
- ¼ cup fresh cranberries
- ¼ teaspoon ground cinnamon
- ¼ cup uncooked wheat berries
- ½ teaspoon fresh ginger, grated finely
- ½ teaspoon canola oil
- 2 drops liquid stevia
- ½ pear, cored and thinly sliced
- ½ teaspoon lemon zest, grated finely

Preparation:
1. Boil water and wheat berries in a pan over medium-high heat and simmer for about 30 minutes.
2. Meanwhile, heat oil in a skillet and cook pear slices in it for about four minutes.
3. Add ginger and cranberries and cook for about two minutes.
4. Stir in wheat berries mixture, lemon zest and cinnamon and cook for about two minutes.
5. Take out, serve and enjoy!

Serving Suggestions: Garnish with whipped cream before serving.
Variation Tip: You can add applesauce to enhance taste.
Nutritional Information per Serving:
Calories: 67 | Fat: 1.4g | Sat Fat: 0.1g | Carbohydrates: 12.9g | Fiber: 2g | Sugar: 4g | Protein: 1.2g

Pistachio Overnight Oats

Prep Time: 10 minutes
Cook Time: 4 hours
Serves: 1
Ingredients:
- ½ cup rolled oats
- 1 tablespoon chia seeds
- ½ cup fat-free milk
- ¼ cup nonfat plain Greek yogurt
- ¼ teaspoon vanilla extract
- ¼ teaspoon ground cinnamon
- 1 teaspoon honey
- ½ cup apple, washed, unpeeled, chopped
- 1 tablespoon unsalted pistachios for serving

Preparation:
1. Mix the oats, yogurt, seeds, milk, spices, vanilla, sweetener and fruit in a jar and stir to combine.
2. Cover and put in the refrigerator for at least 4 hours or overnight.
3. When you are ready to serve, stir and add additional milk if the oats are too thick.
4. Serve.

Serving Suggestion: Top with pistachios.
Variation Tip: Substitute honey with maple syrup.
Nutritional Information per Serving:
Calories 410 | Fat 10 g | Sodium 81 mg | Carbs 57 g | Fiber 10 g | Sugar 22 g | Protein 20 g

Mushroom Shallot Frittata

Prep Time: 10 minutes
Cook Time: 20 minutes
Serves: 4
Ingredients:
- 1 tablespoon butter
- 4 shallots, chopped
- ½ pound mushrooms, diced
- 2 teaspoons parsley, diced
- 3 eggs
- 1 teaspoon dried thyme
- Black pepper to taste
- 5 egg whites
- 1 tablespoon Half and Half milk
- ¼ cup parmesan cheese, grated

Preparation:
1. Preheat the oven to 350°F.
2. Heat a skillet greased with butter on medium heat.
3. Add the shallots to sauté for 5 minutes until golden brown.
4. Stir in the parsley, thyme, mushroom, and black pepper.
5. Beat the eggs with the parmesan, egg whites, and milk in a bowl.
6. Pour this mixture into the mushrooms.
7. Cook for 2 minutes, then bake it for 15 minutes.
8. Slice and serve.

Serving Suggestion: Serve the frittata with a glass of raspberry smoothie.
Variation Tip: Add chopped kale to the frittata.
Nutritional Information per Serving:
Calories 204 | Fat 13g |Sodium 32mg | Carbs 31g | Fiber 3g | Sugar 4g | Protein 7.6g

Greek Yogurt Parfait with Granola

Prep Time: 10 minutes
Cook Time: 25 minutes
Serves: 5
Ingredients:
• 5 cups nonfat plain Greek yogurt
• 1 tablespoon ground cinnamon
• 10 tablespoons Super simple granola or store-bought
• 2½ cups fresh berries (any kind), sliced if large
Preparation:
1. In a medium bowl, stir together the Greek yogurt and cinnamon.
2. Evenly divide the yogurt among 5 storage containers.
3. Distribute 2 tablespoons of granola and ½ cup of fresh berries to each container.
Serving Suggestion: Garnish with mint leaves.
Variation Tip: Feel free to swap in or add pecans, cashews, or pistachios to the granola.
Nutritional Information per Serving:
Calories 265| Fat 7g | Sodium 113mg | Carbs 26g | Fiber 6g | Sugar 10g | Protein 27g

Greek Yogurt Oat Pancakes

Prep Time: 10 minutes
Cook Time: 10 minutes
Serves: 2
Ingredients:
• 6 egg whites
• 1 cup rolled oats
• 1 cup plain nonfat Greek yogurt
• 1 medium banana, peeled and sliced
• 1 teaspoon ground cinnamon
• 1 teaspoon baking powder
Preparation:
1. Blend all of the listed ingredients using a blender.
2. Warm a griddle over medium heat. Spray the skillet with non-stick cooking spray.
3. Put ⅓ cup of the mixture or batter onto the griddle.
4. Allow to cook and flip when bubbles on the top burst, about 5 minutes.
5. Cook again within a minute until golden brown.
6. Repeat with the remaining batter.
7. Divide between two serving plates and enjoy.

Serving Suggestion: Serve with a dollop of maple syrup.
Variation Tip: Substitute the egg whites with ¾ cup liquid egg whites.
Nutritional Information per Serving:
Calories 318| Fat 4 g | Sodium 467 mg | Carbs 47 g | Fiber 6 g | Sugar 13 g | Protein 28 g

Nuts and Oats Granola

Prep Time: 15 minutes
Cook Time: 30 minutes
Serves: 13
Ingredients:
• 2 tablespoons unsweetened applesauce
• 2 tablespoons canola oil
• ¾ teaspoon organic vanilla extract
• 3 cups rolled oats
• ½ cup unsalted almonds
• ¼ cup unsweetened coconut, shredded
• 1 cup bran flakes
• ½ cup unsalted walnuts, chopped
• ½ cup raisins
Preparation:

1. Preheat the baking oven to 325° F and lightly grease a baking dish.
2. Add oil, applesauce and vanilla extract in a pan and cook for about five minutes over low heat.
3. Add in all the other ingredients except raisins and stir well.
4. Transfer the mixture in the baking sheet and bake for about 25 minutes.
5. Take out and set aside to cool.
6. Stir in raisins and serve.
Serving Suggestions: Serve with banana slices on the top.
Variation Tip: Applesauce can be replaced with honey.
Nutritional Information per Serving:
Calories: 176 | Fat: 8.9g | Sat Fat: 1.3g | Carbohydrates: 21.6g | Fiber: 3.6g | Sugar: 4.6g | Protein: 4.5g

Brown Rice Porridge

Prep Time: 10 minutes
Cook Time: 8 minutes
Serves: 4
Ingredients:
• 3 cups cooked brown rice
• 1 ¾ cups nonfat or low-fat milk
• 2 tablespoons lightly packed brown sugar
• 4 dried apricots, chopped
• 1 medium apple, cored and diced
• ¾ teaspoon ground cinnamon
• ¾ teaspoon vanilla extract
Preparation:
1. Combine the rice, milk, sugar, apricots, apple and cinnamon in a medium saucepan.
2. Boil it on medium heat, lower the heat down slightly and cook within 2 to 3 minutes.
3. Turn it off, then stir in the vanilla extract.
4. Serve warm.
Serving Suggestion: Garnish with sliced strawberries.
Variation Tip: Feel free to use coconut milk.
Nutritional Information per Serving:
Calories 260 | Fat 2 g | Sodium 50 mg | Carbs 57 g | Fiber 4 g | Sugar 22 g | Protein 7 g

Pear-Cauliflower Porridge

Prep Time: 10 minutes
Cook Time: 20 minutes
Serves: 3
Ingredients:
• 1 cup shredded pear
• ½ teaspoon organic vanilla extract
• ¼ cup cauliflower rice
• ¼ cup unsweetened coconut, shredded
• ½ cup fat-free milk
Preparation:

1. Add pear, vanilla extract, cauliflower rice, coconut and fat-free milk in a pan. Mix properly.
2. Simmer for about 20 minutes over medium-high heat and take out.
3. Serve and enjoy!
Serving Suggestions: You can serve with pear slices on the top.
Variation Tip: Strawberry can be added to enhance taste.
Nutritional Information per Serving:
Calories: 88 | Fat: 2.7g | Sat Fat: 2.1g | Carbohydrates: 14.4g | Fiber: 2.5g | Sugar: 8.1g | Protein: 2.2g

Zucchini Pancakes

Prep Time: 5 minutes
Cook Time: 23 minutes
Serves: 2
Ingredients:
• 1 tablespoon ground flax seeds
• ½ Jalapeno pepper, finely chopped
• ½ teaspoon olive oil
• ½ cup water
• ½ cup chopped scallion
• 1½ zucchinis, grated finely
Preparation:
1. Mix water and flax seeds in a bowl. Mix well.
2. Meanwhile, heat oil in a non-stick skillet and cook Jalapeno pepper and zucchinis in it for about two minutes. Stirring occasionally.
3. Take out the mixture in a bowl and set aside to cool.
4. Now, add flax seeds and scallion in zucchini mixture and mix well.
5. Preheat the greased griddle and pour ¼ of the zucchini mixture in it.
6. Cook for two minutes per side and repeat the process with remaining mixture.
7. Serve and enjoy!
Serving Suggestions: Serve with lemon wedges.
Variation Tip: Use white pepper to enhance taste.
Nutritional Information per Serving:
Calories: 124 | Fat: 3.3g | Sat Fat: 0.5g | Carbohydrates: 21.1g | Fiber: 7.6g | Sugar: 10.1g | Protein: 7.7g

Banana Almond Yogurt

Prep Time: 10 minutes
Cook Time: 1 minute
Serves: 1
Ingredients:
• 1 tablespoon raw, crunchy, unsalted almond butter
• ¾ cup low-fat plain Greek yogurt
• ¼ cup uncooked old-fashioned oats
• ½ large banana, sliced
• ⅛ teaspoon ground cinnamon
Preparation:
1. Soften the almond butter in the microwave for 15 seconds.
2. Scoop the yogurt into a bowl, and stir in the almond butter, oats and banana.
3. Serve and enjoy
Serving Suggestion: Sprinkle cinnamon on top.
Variation Tip: Feel free to add in berries of your liking.
Nutritional Information per Serving:
Calories 337| Fat 12 g | Sodium 65 mg | Carbs 48 g | Fiber 7 g | Sugar 11 g | Protein 25 g

Banana Almond Pancakes

Prep Time: 10 minutes
Cook Time: 3 minutes
Serves: 1
Ingredients:
• 1 medium banana, sliced
• 2 large eggs
• 2 tablespoon almond meal/flour
• 2 tablespoon quick oats
• 1 teaspoon almond butter
• ½ teaspoon baking powder
• ¼ cup raspberries washed and drained
Preparation:
1. Combine the banana, eggs, oats, almond butter, almond meal/flour and baking powder in a high-powered blender and process until smooth.
2. Coat a pan with cooking spray and set over medium heat.

3. Pour 2 tablespoon batter onto the pan and let cook for about 1 minute.
4. Flip and cook on the other side for about 1 minute more until lightly browned and firm.
5. Serve
Serving Suggestion: Top with fresh berries.
Variation Tip: Although this recipe is written for one, you can easily double or triple the recipe to fit your household.
Nutritional Information per Serving:
Calories 414 | Fat 21 g | Sodium 146 mg | Carbs 43 g | Fiber 8 g | Sugar 17 g | Protein 19 g

Baked Carrot Oatmeal

Prep Time: 15 minutes
Cook Time: 37 minutes
Servings: 8
Ingredients:
• 1½ teaspoons ground cinnamon
• 2 teaspoons organic vanilla extract
• 2¼ cups rolled oats
• ¼ cup applesauce, unsweetened
• 1½ teaspoons fresh ginger, finely grated
• 1½ teaspoons organic baking powder
• 2½ cups unsweetened almond milk
• ½ cup unsalted walnuts, chopped
• ¼ cup raisins
• Pinch of salt
• 2½ cups carrots, peeled and shredded
Preparation:
1. Preheat the oven to 375°F and lightly grease a casserole dish.
2. Mix the oats, baking powder, cinnamon, and salt in a large bowl.
3. Mix the applesauce, almond milk, and vanilla extract in another bowl.
4. Add the oats mixture to the almond milk mixture and mix until well combined.
5. Fold in the carrots and ginger.
6. Put the mixture into the prepared casserole dish.
7. Top evenly with raisins and walnuts.
8. Bake for about 37 minutes, then serve warm.
Serving Suggestion: Top with chopped pecans before serving.
Variation Tip: Cinnamon can be added to enhance the taste.
Nutritional Information per Serving:
Calories: 301|Fat: 9.3g|Sat Fat: 2.3g|Carbohydrates: 46.7g|Fiber: 7.7g|Sugar: 5.9g|Protein: 9.7g

Raspberry Smoothie Bowl

Prep Time: 10 minutes
Serves: 4
Ingredients:
- 4 cups frozen blueberries
- 1 cup unsweetened almond milk
- 4 drops liquid stevia
- 4 tablespoons unsweetened protein powder
- ½ cup fat-free plain Greek yogurt

Preparation:
1. Add blueberries in a blender and blend well.
2. Add all the remaining ingredients and blend until a smooth mixture is formed.
3. Pour in bowls and serve with a smile.

Serving Suggestions: Top with blueberries before serving.
Variation Tip: You can use coconut milk instead of almond milk.
Nutritional Information per Serving:
Calories: 220 | Fat: 2.4g | Sat Fat: 0.1g | Carbohydrates: 22.8g | Fiber: 3.8g | Sugar: 15.5g | Protein: 28.4g

Apple and Millet Muffins

Prep Time: 5 minutes
Cook Time: 20 minutes
Serves: 6
Ingredients:
- 1 apple, cored and grated
- ½ cup uncooked millet
- ½ cup raisins
- ½ cup sunflower seeds

- 1 tablespoon fresh lemon juice
- ¼ tablespoon fresh lemon zest, grated finely
- ½ cup fresh apple juice

Preparation:
1. Preheat the baking oven to 350° F and grease six muffin tins.
2. Meanwhile, add all the ingredients except apple juice in a large bowl and mix well.
3. Transfer the mixture in muffin tins and drizzle each muffin tin with apple juice.
4. Cover muffin tins with a foil and bake for about 20 minutes.
5. Take out and set aside to cool.
6. Serve and enjoy!

Serving Suggestions: Serve with apple slices on the top.
Variation Tip: Cardamom can be added to enhance taste.
Nutritional Information per Serving:
Calories: 151 | Fat: 2.8g | Sat Fat: 0.3g | Carbohydrates: 30g | Fiber: 3.2g | Sugar: 13.2g | Protein: 3.2g

Oat Waffles

Prep Time: 5 minutes
Cook Time: 10 minutes
Serves: 1
Ingredients:
- ½ cup rolled oats
- 2 egg whites
- ¼ teaspoon stevia
- ¼ teaspoon organic vanilla extract
- ¼ teaspoon organic baking powder
- ¼ cup water
- ¾ teaspoon olive oil

Preparation:

1. Add everything in a food processor and pulse well.
2. Preheat the waffle iron and lightly grease it.
3. Pour the mixture in the waffle iron and cook for about five minutes.
4. Take out and serve warm.

Serving Suggestions: Top with unsweetened applesauce before serving.
Variation Tip: Stevia can be omitted.
Nutritional Information per Serving:
Calories: 224 | Fat: 6.3g | Sat Fat: 1g | Carbohydrates: 28.9g | Fiber: 4.2g | Sugar: 1g | Protein: 12.6g

Scrambled Eggs

Prep Time: 5 minutes
Cook Time: 8 minutes
Serves: 3
Ingredients:
- 1 tablespoon unsalted margarine
- 1 tablespoon chopped chives
- ½ red onion, finely chopped
- ½ Jalapeno pepper, seeded and chopped
- 6 eggs, lightly beaten
- Black pepper, to taste

Preparation:

1. Heat margarine in a large skillet and sauté onion and Jalapeno pepper in it for about five minutes.
2. Add in eggs and pepper and cook for about three minutes. Stirring continuously.
3. Take out and immediately stir in cheese and chives.
4. Serve and enjoy!

Serving Suggestions: Top with chopped mint leaves before serving.
Variation Tip: Add olives to enhance taste.
Nutritional Information per Serving:
Calories: 168 | Fat: 12.6g | Sat Fat: 3.4g | Carbohydrates: 2.6g | Fiber: 0.5g | Sugar: 1.6g | Protein: 11.4g

Quinoa Bread

Prep Time: 15 minutes
Cook Time: 1 hour
Servings: 10
Ingredients:
- 1 teaspoon baking soda

- 2 cups uncooked quinoa, rinsed
- ¼ teaspoon ground cinnamon
- 1 tablespoon fresh lemon juice
- 1 teaspoon organic baking powder
- 3 tablespoons unsalted margarine, melted
- 2 cups almond milk, unsweetened
- 1 cup oat flour
- Pinch of salt
- 1 tablespoon black sesame seeds

Preparation:
1. Preheat the oven to 400°F and lightly grease a loaf pan.
2. Put the quinoa in the food processor and pulse until a flour-like texture forms.
3. Shift the quinoa flour into a large bowl.
4. Add the oat flour, baking soda, baking powder, cinnamon, and salt and mix well.
5. Add the milk, margarine, and lemon juice to another bowl and beat until well combined.
6. Add the milk mixture into the flour mixture and mix until well combined.
7. Place the mixture into the prepared loaf pan evenly and sprinkle evenly with sesame seeds.
8. Using a piece of foil, loosely cover the loaf pan and bake for about 30 minutes.
9. Remove the foil and bake for another 30 minutes.
10. Remove the loaf pan from the oven and place it onto a wire rack to cool for about 10 minutes.
11. Cut the bread into desired-sized slices and serve.

Serving Suggestion: Serve with a topping of pecans.
Variation Tip: You can substitute the almond milk with coconut milk.
Nutritional Information per Serving:
Calories: 206|Fat: 7.3g|Sat Fat: 2.1g|Carbohydrates: 29.1g|Fiber: 3.6g|Sugar: 0g|Protein: 6.4g

Baked French Toast

Prep Time: 10 minutes
Cook Time: 8 minutes
Servings: 4
Ingredients:
- 1¼ cups unsweetened almond milk
- 4 drops liquid stevia
- 2 tablespoons olive oil
- 4 eggs
- 4 (¾-inch thick) white bread slices, trimmed and sliced diagonally

Preparation:
1. Preheat the oven to 400°F and lightly grease a baking sheet.

2. In a bowl, add the almond milk and eggs and beat lightly.

3. Dip each bread slice evenly into the egg mixture.

4. Heat the oil in a skillet and cook the bread slices for about 1 minute on each side over medium heat.

5. Layer the slices onto the baking sheet and bake for about 4 minutes.

6. Serve warm.

Serving Suggestion: Serve topped with whipped cream.

Variation Tip: You can also use coconut milk.

Nutritional Information per Serving:
Calories: 202|Fat: 13.3g|Sat Fat: 3g|Carbohydrates: 13.6g|Fiber: 0.9g|Sugar: 1.4g|Protein: 7.8g

Banana Bread

Prep Time: 10 minutes
Cook Time: 1 hour
Servings: 12
Ingredients:

- ¼ teaspoon ground cardamom
- ⅓ cup fat-free milk
- 1½ cups whole-wheat flour
- 2 eggs
- 2 teaspoons organic vanilla extract
- Pinch of salt
- ¼ cup canola oil
- 1 teaspoon powdered stevia
- 1 cup ripe banana, peeled and mashed
- ½ cup unsalted walnuts, chopped

Preparation:

1. Preheat the oven to 350°F and lightly grease a loaf pan.

2. Mix the flour, baking soda, stevia, cardamom, and salt in a bowl.

3. Add the eggs, banana, milk, oil, and vanilla extract to another bowl and beat until well combined.

4. Add the banana mixture to the flour mixture and mix until just combined. Fold in the walnuts.

5. Put the mixture into the prepared loaf pan.

6. Bake for about 1 hour in the preheated oven.

7. Tip the bread out onto a wire rack to cool before slicing. Cut the bread into desired-sized slices and serve.

Serving Suggestion: Serve topped with cream cheese frosting.

Variation Tip: You can use pecans instead of walnuts.

Nutritional Information per Serving:
Calories: 155|Fat: 8.5g|Sat Fat: 1.4g|Carbohydrates: 15.8g|Fiber: 1.1g|Sugar: 2.1g|Protein: 4.1g

Cherry Pancakes

Prep Time: 25 minutes
Cook Time: 5 minutes
Servings: 4
Ingredients:

- ⅛ teaspoon ground cinnamon
- 1 teaspoon margarine, unsalted
- 3 eggs
- 2 cups fresh sweet cherries, pitted and halved
- Pinch of salt
- 1 teaspoon organic vanilla extract
- 1 tablespoon unsalted margarine, melted
- ½ cup whole-wheat pastry flour
- ½ cup fat-free milk
- ¼ cup unsalted almonds, chopped

Preparation:

1. Preheat the oven to 450°F.

2. Add 1 teaspoon of margarine to a 10-inch ovenproof skillet and place the skillet into the preheated oven.

3. In a bowl, mix the flour, cinnamon, and salt. Add the eggs, milk, melted margarine, and vanilla to another bowl and beat until well combined.

4. Add the egg mixture to the flour mixture and mix until well combined.

5. Remove the skillet from the oven and tilt it to spread the melted margarine evenly.

6. Place the cherries in the bottom of the skillet in a single layer. Place the flour mixture over the cherries evenly and top with the almonds.

7. Bake for about 20 minutes.

8. Remove from the oven and set aside to cool for at least 5 minutes before slicing. Cut into 4 equal-sized wedges and serve.

Serving Suggestion: Serve along with a cup of tea.

Variation Tip: You can substitute cherries with blueberries.

Nutritional Information per Serving:
Calories: 268|Fat: 14g|Sat Fat: 3g|Carbohydrates: 9g|Fiber: 1g|Sugar: 4g|Protein: 26g

Eggs on Toast

Prep Time: 10 minutes
Cook Time: 3 minutes
Servings: 2
Ingredients:
• 2 whole-wheat bread slices
• Black pepper, to taste
• 2 teaspoons low-fat parmesan cheese, grated
• 2 large eggs
Preparation:
1. Using a biscuit cutter, press a hole in the center of each bread slice.
2. Heat a greased non-stick skillet over medium-low heat.
3. Arrange a bread slice in the skillet and carefully crack an egg in the center of the hole.
4. Cook for about 45 seconds. Season with black pepper and carefully flip the slice.
5. Cook for about 1 minute, then repeat with the remaining bread slice and egg.
Serving Suggestion: Sprinkle with parmesan cheese and serve.
Variation Tip: You can also add any other low-fat cheese.
Nutritional Information per Serving:
Calories: 138|Fat: 6.1g|Sat Fat: 1.5g|Carbohydrates: 10.8g|Fiber: 1.7g|Sugar: 1.8g|Protein: 9.9g

Baked Spinach and Eggs

Prep Time: 10 minutes
Cook Time: 22 minutes
Servings: 4
Ingredients:
• 4 eggs
• 7 cups fresh baby spinach
• Black pepper, to taste
• Pinch of salt
• 4 tablespoons water
• 3 tablespoons feta cheese, crumbled
Preparation:

1. Preheat the oven to 400°F and lightly grease 2 small baking dishes.
2. Add the spinach and water over medium heat to a large-sized pan and cook for about 4 minutes.
3. Remove the pan from the heat and drain the excess water completely.
4. Divide the spinach evenly into the prepared baking dishes.
5. Carefully crack 2 eggs over the spinach in each baking dish.
6. Season with salt and black pepper and top evenly with feta cheese.
7. Put the baking dishes in the oven and bake for about 18 minutes.
8. Remove from the oven and set aside for about 5 minutes before serving.
Serving Suggestion: Serve alongside a cup of freshly-brewed tea.
Variation Tip: You can also use goat's cheese instead of feta cheese.
Nutritional Information per Serving:
Calories: 94|Fat: 6.1g|Sat Fat: 1.3g|Carbohydrates: 2.6g|Fiber: 1.2g|Sugar: 0.9g|Protein: 8g

French Toast

Prep Time: 10 minutes
Cook Time: 32 minutes
Servings: 4
Ingredients:
• $1^1/_3$ cups egg whites
• 2 teaspoons powdered stevia
• ½ cup fresh strawberries
• $1^1/_3$ cups fat-free milk
• 8 whole-wheat bread slices
Preparation:
1. Put the egg whites, milk, and stevia in a shallow bowl and beat well.
2. Dip the bread slices evenly in the egg mixture one at a time.
3. Heat a large greased non-stick skillet over medium heat.
4. Add the bread slices, one at a time, and cook for about 2 minutes per side.
5. Serve warm topped with strawberries.
Serving Suggestion: Serve with whipped cream.
Variation Tip: You can omit stevia from this recipe.
Nutritional Information per Serving:
Calories: 201|Fat: 1.9g|Sat Fat: 0.2g|Carbohydrates: 26.6g|Fiber: 3.8g|Sugar: 8.2g|Protein: 18g

Spaghetti Frittata

Prep Time: 10 minutes
Cook Time: 10 minutes
Servings: 5
Ingredients:
- 2½ cups fat-free milk
- 4 large eggs
- 2 teaspoons olive oil
- 2 tablespoons fresh basil leaves, chopped
- Black pepper, to taste
- ⅓ cup scallions, chopped
- 2 ounces part-skim mozzarella cheese, shredded
- 2 large egg whites
- 2½ cups whole-wheat spaghetti, cooked

Preparation:
1. Mix the eggs, egg whites, and black pepper in a bowl and beat until well combined. Set aside.
2. Heat the oil in a medium non-stick skillet and cook the spaghetti for about 2 minutes over medium heat.
3. Top evenly with the egg mixture and sprinkle with the scallions, cheese, and basil.
4. Cook for about 8 minutes, then place onto a large plate.
5. Cut into 4 equal-sized wedges and serve.
Serving Suggestion: Serve garnished with parsley.
Variation Tip: You can use any type of spaghetti you prefer.
Nutritional Information per Serving:
Calories: 225|Fat: 9.9g|Sat Fat: 2.5g|Carbohydrates: 17.7g|Fiber: 2.2g|Sugar: 13g|Protein: 15.2g

Tofu and Veggie Hash

Prep Time: 15 minutes
Cook Time: 15 minutes
Servings: 2
Ingredients:
- 1 small bell pepper, seeded and chopped finely
- ½ tablespoon canola oil
- 1½ cup firm tofu, pressed, drained, and crumbled
- 1 small onion, chopped finely
- Pinch of cayenne pepper
- 1 tablespoon fresh parsley leaves, chopped
- Pinch of salt
- 1 cup cherry tomatoes, chopped finely
- Pinch of ground turmeric

Preparation:
1. Heat the oil over medium heat in a skillet and sauté the onion and bell pepper for about 5 minutes.
2. Add the tomatoes and cook for about 2 minutes.
3. Add the tofu and spices and cook for about 8 minutes.
4. Garnish with parsley leaves and serve.
Serving Suggestion: Serve sprinkled with the extra spices.
Variation Tip: You can add veggies of your choice.
Nutritional Information per Serving:
Calories: 214|Fat: 11.8g|Sat Fat: 4g|Carbohydrates: 14.7g|Fiber: 4.5g|Sugar: 8g|Protein: 17.3g

Apple Crepes

Prep Time: 15 minutes
Cook Time: 24 minutes
Servings: 4
Ingredients:
- Pinch of salt
- 1½ cups whole-wheat flour
- 1½ cups fat-free milk
- ½ teaspoon powdered stevia
- 2 tablespoons unsalted margarine, melted and cooled
- 2 apples, peeled, cored, and sliced thinly
- 3 large eggs, beaten

Preparation:
1. Sift together the flour, stevia, and salt in a large bowl.
2. Make a well in the center of the flour mixture.
3. Add the beaten egg to the well and mix well. Slowly add the milk, mixing again.
4. Add the margarine and mix until well combined.
5. Cover the bowl and set it aside for about 2 hours at room temperature.
6. Heat a non-stick skillet over medium-low heat.
7. Add about ¼ cup of the mixture and tilt the pan to spread it evenly in the bottom of the skillet.
8. Place about 8 apple slices evenly over the crepe mixture and cook for about 2 minutes.
9. Carefully flip the crepe and cook it for another 2 minutes.

10. Repeat with the remaining mixture and serve warm.
Serving Suggestion: Serve with applesauce.
Variation Tip: You can also make banana crepes with this recipe.
Nutritional Information per Serving:
Calories: 367|Fat: 10.6g|Sat Fat: 2.9g|Carbohydrates: 56g|Fiber: 4g|Sugar: 16.5g|Protein: 12.9g

Microwaved Egg Scramble

Prep Time: 10 minutes
Cook Time: 1 minute 30 seconds
Servings: 2
Ingredients:
• 4 egg whites
• ¼ cup fat-free milk
• Black pepper, to taste
• ¼ cup fresh mushrooms, finely chopped
• 2 eggs
Preparation:
1. Add the milk, eggs, and egg whites to a bowl and beat until well combined.
2. Stir in the mushrooms.
3. Divide the egg mixture evenly into 2 greased mugs and microwave on high power for about 45 seconds.
4. Remove the mugs from the microwave and stir well.
5. Place the mugs back into the microwave, cook on high power for about 45 seconds more, and then serve immediately.
Serving Suggestion: Serve with toast.
Variation Tip: You can also make this egg scramble on the stove.
Nutritional Information per Serving:
Calories: 110|Fat: 4.5g|Sat Fat: 0.5g|Carbohydrates: 2.6g|Fiber: 0.1g|Sugar: 2.5g|Protein: 14g

Bell Pepper and Turkey Muffins

Prep Time: 10 minutes
Cook Time: 20 minutes
Serves: 4
Ingredients:
• 4 eggs
• 1 tablespoon water
• ½ cup bell peppers, seeded and chopped
• ½ cup chopped onion
• ½ tablespoon fresh parsley, chopped
• ¼ tablespoon red pepper flakes, crushed
• 4 ounces cooked turkey, finely chopped
• Black pepper, to taste
Preparation:
1. Preheat the oven to 350° F and grease four muffin tins.
2. Meanwhile, add water, eggs, red pepper flakes, parsley and black pepper in a bowl. Mix well.
3. Add in turkey, onion and bell peppers and mix properly.
4. Pour the mixture in muffin tins and bake for about 20 minutes.
5. Take out and set aside to cool.
6. Serve and enjoy!
Serving Suggestions: Garnish with chopped cilantro before serving.
Variation Tip: Replace black pepper with white pepper.
Nutritional Information per Serving:
Calories: 123 | Fat: 5.9g | Sat Fat: 1.8g | Carbohydrates: 3.1g | Fiber: 0.6g | Sugar: 1.7g | Protein: 14.2g

Quinoa Porridge

Prep Time: 5 minutes
Cook Time: 20 minutes
Serves: 2
Ingredients:
- 1 cup unsweetened soy milk
- ½ cup uncooked quinoa, rinsed
- ¼ tablespoons organic vanilla extract
- ½ date, pitted and chopped finely
- ½ cups sliced banana

Preparation:
1. Add soymilk, quinoa and vanilla extract in a pan and cook for about 20 minutes.
2. Stir in date and take out.
3. Top with banana slices and serve.

Serving Suggestions: Top with dates before serving.
Variation Tip: Cinnamon can also be added to enhance taste.
Nutritional Information per Serving:
Calories: 267 | Fat: 4.9g | Sat Fat: 0.6g |
Carbohydrates: 45.3g | Fiber: 4.9g | Sugar: 11g |
Protein: 10.5g

Rhubarb Pecan Muffins

Prep Time: 15 minutes
Cook Time: 30 minutes
Serves: 6
Ingredients:
- 1 cup all-purpose flour
- 1 cup whole-wheat flour
- ½ cup sugar
- 1½ teaspoons baking powder
- ½ teaspoon baking soda
- ½ teaspoon salt
- 2 egg whites
- 2 tablespoons canola oil
- 2 tablespoons unsweetened applesauce
- 2 teaspoons grated orange peel
- ¾ cup orange juice
- 1¼ cup rhubarb, chopped
- 2 tablespoons pecans, chopped

Preparation:
1. Preheat the oven to 350°F. Layer a muffin pan with muffin paper.
2. Combine the flours with the baking soda, baking powder, and sugar in a bowl.
3. Whisk the egg whites with the orange peel, orange juice, applesauce, and canola oil in a separate bowl.
4. Add the wet mixture to the dry ingredients and mix well until smooth.
5. Fold in the chopped rhubarb, then divide the mixture into the muffin cups.
6. Top the batter with a ½ teaspoon of chopped pecans.
7. Bake for 30 minutes, then allow the muffins to cool.
8. Serve.

Serving Suggestion Serve the muffins with a glass of kiwi smoothie.
Variation Tip: Drizzle chocolate syrup over the muffins.
Nutritional Information per Serving:
Calories 147 | Fat 15g |Sodium 31mg | Carbs 22g |
Fiber 4g | Sugar 1g | Protein 4.1g

Whole-Wheat Pretzels

Prep Time: 15 minutes
Cook Time: 17 minutes
Serves: 6
Ingredients:
- 1 sachet active dry yeast
- 2 teaspoons brown sugar
- ½ teaspoon salt
- 1½ cups warm water
- 1 cup bread flour
- 3 cups whole-wheat flour
- 1 tablespoon olive oil
- ½ cup wheat gluten
- Cooking spray
- ¼ cup baking soda
- ¼ cup egg substitute
- 1 tablespoon of sesame seeds

Preparation:
1. Mix the yeast with the salt, sugar, and water in a bowl and let it rest for 5 minutes.

2. Combine the flours with the gluten and olive oil in a processor.
3. Mix in the yeast mixture and knead the dough until smooth.
4. Cover the dough in a bowl with a plastic sheet and keep it in a warm place for 1 hour until the dough has risen.
5. Preheat the oven to 450°F.
6. Punch down on the dough and divide it into 14 pieces.
7. Roll each piece into long ropes and make a pretzel shape out of each.
8. Boil 10 cups of water with ¼ cup baking soda in a pot. Place the pretzels in the water.
9. Cook each pretzel for 30 seconds, then immediately transfer them to a baking pan lined with parchment paper using a slotted spoon.
10. Brush each pretzel with whisked egg whites and sprinkle sesame, sunflower, and poppy seeds on top.
11. Bake them for 15 minutes.
12. Serve.
Serving Suggestion: Serve the pretzels with a glass of strawberry smoothie.
Variation Tip: Drizzle chocolate syrup over the pretzels.
Nutritional Information per Serving:
Calories 218 | Fat 22g |Sodium 50mg | Carbs 22g | Fiber 0.7g | Sugar 1g |Protein 2.3g

Raspberry Chocolate Scones

Prep Time: 15 minutes
Cook Time: 10 minutes
Serves: 6
Ingredients:
• 1 cup whole-wheat pastry flour
• 1 cup all-purpose flour
• 1 tablespoon baking powder
• ¼ teaspoon baking soda
• ⅓ cup buttery spread
• ½ cup fresh raspberries
• ¼ cup miniature chocolate chips
• 2 tablespoons plain fat-free yogurt
• 2 tablespoons honey
• ½ teaspoon sugar
• ¼ teaspoon cinnamon
Preparation:
1. Preheat the oven to 400°F.
2. Combine the flours with the baking soda and baking powder in a mixing bowl.
3. Cut the butter into the dry mixture until it forms a crumbly mixture.
4. Fold in the chocolate chips and berries.

5. Pour in the honey and yogurt, then stir the mixture gently to form a crumbly batter.
6. Knead the batter into a dough ball on a surface, then spread it into a ½-inch thick circle.
7. Slice the circle into 12 wedges, then arrange them on a greased baking tray.
8. Sprinkle the sugar and cinnamon mixture on top.
9. Bake for 12 minutes.
10. Serve and enjoy.
Serving Suggestion: Serve the meal with a glass of spirulina smoothie.
Variation Tip: Drizzle maple syrup over the scones.
Nutritional Information per Serving:
Calories 149 | Fat 12g |Sodium 102mg | Carbs 26g | Fiber 4g | Sugar 1.3g |Protein 4.2g

Apple Omelet

Prep Time: 10 minutes
Cook Time: 10 minutes
Servings: 2
Ingredients:
• ¼ teaspoon ground cinnamon
• 3 teaspoons olive oil, divided
• ⅛ teaspoon organic vanilla extract
• 1 large green apple, cored and sliced thinly
• Pinch of salt
• 1 teaspoon unsweetened applesauce
• 4 eggs
Preparation:
1. Put 1 teaspoon of oil in a non-stick frying pan. Cook the apple slices, cinnamon, and nutmeg for about 5 minutes over medium-low heat, turning once.
2. Meanwhile, add the eggs, vanilla extract, and salt to a bowl and beat until fluffy.
3. Add the remaining olive oil to the skillet and let it heat up.
4. Place the egg mixture evenly over the apple slices and cook for about 4 minutes.
5. Carefully turn the skillet over a serving plate and fold the omelet.
Serving Suggestion: Serve with a drizzle of applesauce.
Variation Tip: Use any kind of apple.
Nutritional Information per Serving:
Calories: 185|Fat: 9g|Sat Fat: 2g|Carbohydrates: 16.6g|Fiber: 2.9g|Sugar: 12.6g|Protein: 11.4g

Zucchini Bread

Prep Time: 25 minutes
Cook Time: 50 minutes
Serves: 18 (2 loaves)
Ingredients
- ¼ cup egg whites
- 1 cup canola oil
- ½ cup unsweetened applesauce
- ½ cup sugar
- 2 tsp. vanilla extract
- 1¼ cups all-purpose (plain) flour
- 1¼ cups whole-wheat (whole-meal) flour
- 1 tsp. baking powder
- 1 tsp. baking soda
- 3 tsp. ground cinnamon
- 2 cups shredded zucchini
- ½ cup chopped walnuts
- 1½ cups crushed, unsweetened pineapple

Preparation
1. Heat the oven to 350°F. Lightly coat two 9 x 5-inch loaf pans with cooking spray.
2. In a large bowl, add the egg whites, canola oil, applesauce, sugar, and vanilla. Using an electric mixer, beat the mixture on low speed until thick and foamy.
3. In a small bowl, stir together the flours. Set ½ cup aside. Add the baking powder, baking soda, and cinnamon to the small bowl of flour.
4. Add the flour mixture to the egg white mixture. Using the electric mixer on medium speed, beat until well-blended.
5. Add the zucchini, walnuts, and pineapple and stir until combined. Adjust the consistency of the batter with the remaining ½ cup flour, adding 1 tablespoon at a time. The batter should be thick and not runny.
6. Pour half of the batter into each prepared pan. Bake until a toothpick inserted into the centers of the loaves comes out clean, about 50 minutes.
7. Let the bread cool in the pans on a wire rack for 10 minutes. Turn the loaves out of the pans onto the rack and let cool completely.
Serving Suggestion: Cut each loaf into nine 1-inch slices and serve with tea.
Variation Tip: You can add more nuts of your choice.

Nutritional Information Per Serving:
Calories 141 | Protein 4g | Carbohydrate 22g | Dietary fiber 2g | Sugar 5g | Fat 5g | Sodium 103mg

Buckwheat Pancakes

Prep Time: 10 minutes
Cook Time: 20 minutes
Serves: 6
Ingredients
- 2 egg whites
- 1 tbsp. canola oil
- ½ cup fat-free milk
- ½ cup all-purpose (plain) flour
- ½ cup buckwheat flour
- 1 tbsp. baking powder
- 1 tbsp. sugar
- ½ cup sparkling water
- 3 cups sliced fresh strawberries

Preparation
1. In a small bowl, whisk together the egg whites, canola oil, and milk.
2. In another bowl, combine the flours, baking powder, and sugar. Add the egg white mixture and the sparkling water and stir until slightly moistened.
3. Place a non-stick frying pan or skillet over medium heat. When a drop of water sizzles as it hits the pan, spoon ½ cup pancake batter into the pan. Cook until the top surface of the pancake is covered with bubbles and the edges are lightly browned (about 2 minutes).
4. Turn and cook until the bottom is well-browned and the pancake is cooked through, 1 to 2 minutes longer. Repeat with the remaining pancake batter.
Serving Suggestion: Transfer the pancakes to individual plates. Top each with ½ cup sliced strawberries and serve immediately.
Variation Tip: Instead of maple syrup, top these pancakes with sliced strawberries or other types of fresh fruit such as sliced bananas or peaches.
Nutritional Information Per Serving:
Calories 143 | Protein 5g | Carbohydrate 24g |Dietary fiber 3g | Sugars 2g | Fat 8.2g | Sodium 295mg

Zucchini Frittata

Prep Time: 15 minutes
Cook Time: 16 minutes
Servings: 4
Ingredients:
- $\frac{1}{8}$ teaspoon ground cumin
- 2 large eggs
- Black pepper, to taste
- ½ cup onion, chopped
- 4 egg whites
- 1 tablespoon olive oil
- 2 cups zucchini, sliced thinly
- 3 garlic cloves, minced
- 1 small tomato, chopped
- Pinch of salt
- 2 tablespoons green chili, chopped
- 2 teaspoons fresh parsley, chopped

Preparation:
1. Mix the eggs, egg whites, and spices in a bowl and beat until well combined. Set aside.
2. In a non-stick skillet, heat the oil and sauté the onion for about 2 minutes over medium heat.
3. Add the garlic and green chili and sauté for about 1 minute.
4. Add the zucchini and sauté for about 3 minutes.
5. Sprinkle over the tomato and parsley and top evenly with the egg mixture.
6. Switch the heat to low and cook, covered, for about 10 minutes.
7. Remove from the heat and cut into 4 equal-sized portions to serve.

Serving Suggestion: Serve hot with toasted bagels.
Variation Tip: You can also use some Sichuan red pepper flakes to add spiciness.
Nutritional Information per Serving:
Calories: 108|Fat: 6.2g|Sat Fat: 1.2g|Carbohydrates: 6.9g|Fiber: 1.3g|Sugar: 2.9g|Protein: 8g

Pumpkin Tea Cake

Prep Time: 10 minutes
Cook Time: 55 minutes
Serves: 4
Ingredients:
- 3 tablespoons canola oil
- ½ cup honey
- ¾ cup canned pumpkin puree
- 3 tablespoons brown sugar
- 2 eggs, beaten
- 1 cup whole-wheat flour
- ½ cup all-purpose flour
- 2 tablespoons flaxseed
- ½ teaspoon baking powder
- ½ teaspoon ground allspice
- ½ teaspoon ground cinnamon
- ½ teaspoon ground nutmeg
- ¼ teaspoon ground cloves
- ¼ teaspoon salt
- 2 tablespoons hazelnuts, chopped

Preparation:
1. Grease an 8-inch x 4-inch loaf pan with cooking spray. Preheat the oven to 350°F.
2. Beat the pumpkin puree with the brown sugar, honey, eggs, and canola oil in a mixer.
3. Stir in the flaxseed, allspice, baking powder, flours, cinnamon, cloves, salt, flours, and salt.
4. Mix well until it forms a smooth batter.
5. Transfer this batter to the loaf pan. Top it evenly with hazelnuts.
6. Press the nuts down, then bake the loaf pan for 55 minutes.
7. Allow the bread to cool for 10 minutes.
8. Slice and serve.

Serving Suggestion: Serve the bread with a glass of kale smoothie.
Variation Tip: Add chopped nuts to the cake.
Nutritional Information per Serving:
Calories 166 | Fat 8g |Sodium 146mg | Carbs 28g | Fiber 5g | Sugar 1g | Protein 11.2g

Spinach Omelet

Prep Time: 10 minutes
Cook Time: 15 minutes
Servings: 2
Ingredients:

- ¾ cup chickpea flour
- ½ cup tomato, seeded and chopped finely
- Pinch of salt
- ½ cup water
- 2 tablespoons olive oil
- Black pepper, to taste
- 1¼ cups fresh spinach, chopped finely
- ½ teaspoon cumin seeds
- 1 small green chili, seeded and chopped finely

Preparation:
1. Mix the cumin seeds, salt, and black pepper in a bowl.
2. Slowly add the water and mix until a smooth mixture forms.
3. Add the spinach, tomato, and green chili and mix until well combined.
4. Put 1 tablespoon of oil in a non-stick skillet and cook the spinach mixture over medium heat for about 7 minutes.
5. Put the remaining oil over the omelet, then flip it.
6. Cook for about 5 minutes and serve warm.

Serving Suggestion: Serve over buttered noodles.
Variation Tip: You can also add cayenne pepper to this omelet.

Nutritional Information per Serving:
Calories: 268|Fat: 16.6g|Sat Fat: 6g|Carbohydrates: 22.6g|Fiber: 4.8g|Sugar: 5g|Protein: 8.8g

Slow-Cooked Mediterranean Chicken and Chickpea Soup

Prep Time: 4 hours 20 minutes
Cook Time: 20 minutes
Serves: 6
Ingredients
- 1½ cups dried chickpeas, soaked overnight
- 4 cups water
- 1 large yellow onion, finely chopped
- 1 (15 oz.) can no-salt-added diced tomatoes, preferably fire-roasted
- 2 tbsp. tomato paste
- 4 cloves garlic, finely chopped
- 1 bay leaf
- 4 tsp. ground cumin
- 4 tsp. paprika
- ¼ tsp. cayenne pepper
- ¼ tsp. ground pepper
- 2 lbs. bone-in chicken thighs, skin removed, trimmed
- 1 (14 oz.) can artichoke hearts, drained and quartered
- ¼ cup halved pitted oil-cured olives
- ½ tsp. salt
- ¼ cup chopped fresh parsley or cilantro

Preparation
1. Drain the chickpeas and place them in a 6-quart (or larger) slow cooker. Add 4 cups water, onion, tomatoes and their juice, tomato paste, garlic, bay leaf, cumin, paprika, cayenne, and ground pepper. Stir to combine.
2. Add the chicken.
3. Cover and cook on low for 8 hours or on high for 4 hours.
4. Transfer the chicken to a clean cutting board and let it cool slightly. Discard the bay leaf.
5. Add the artichokes, olives, and salt to the slow cooker and stir to combine.
6. Shred the chicken, discarding the bones. Stir the chicken back into the soup.

Serving Suggestion: Serve topped with parsley (or cilantro).
Variation Tip: Add spices of your choice.
Nutritional Information Per Serving:
Calories 447 | Protein 33.6g | Carbohydrates 43g | Dietary fiber 11.6g | Sugars 8.5g | Fat 15.3g | Sodium 761.8mg

Roasted Root Vegetables With Goat's Cheese Polenta

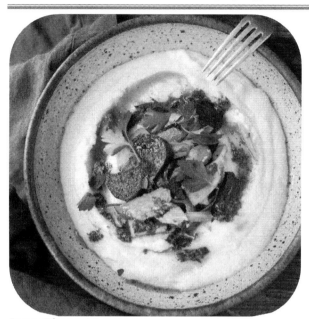

Prep Time: 35 minutes
Cook Time: 25 minutes
Serves: 2
Ingredients
Polenta:
- 2 cups low-sodium vegetable or chicken broth
- ½ cup polenta fine cornmeal or corn grits
- ¼ cup goat's cheese
- 1 tbsp. extra-virgin olive oil or butter
- ¼ tsp. kosher salt
- ¼ tsp. ground pepper
Vegetables:
- 1 tbsp. extra-virgin olive oil or butter
- 1 clove garlic, smashed
- 2 cups roasted root vegetables
- 1 tbsp. torn fresh sage
- 2 tsp. prepared pesto
- Fresh parsley for garnish

Preparation
1. To prepare the polenta: Bring the broth to a boil in a medium saucepan. Reduce the heat to low and gradually add the polenta (or cornmeal or grits), whisking vigorously to avoid clumping. Cover and cook for 10 minutes. Stir, cover, and continue cooking until thickened and creamy, about 10 minutes more. Stir in the goat's cheese, oil (or butter), salt, and pepper.
2. Meanwhile, to prepare the vegetables: Heat the oil (or butter) in a medium skillet over medium heat. Add the garlic and cook, stirring, until fragrant, about 1 minute. Add the roasted vegetables and cook, stirring often, until heated through, 2 to 4 minutes. Stir in the torn sage and cook until fragrant, about 1 minute more.

Serving Suggestion: Serve the vegetables over the polenta, topped with pesto. Garnish with parsley, if desired.
Variation Tip: Add spices of your choice.
Nutritional Information Per Serving:
Calories 442 | Protein 9.1g | Carbohydrates 41.4g | Dietary fiber 7.7g | Sugars 7.7g | Fat 27.7g | Sodium 589.4mg

Turkey Barley Soup

Prep Time: 10 minutes
Cook Time: 20 minutes
Serves: 8
Ingredients:
- 1 tablespoon canola oil
- 5 carrots, chopped
- 1 medium onion, chopped
- ²⁄₃ cup quick-cooking barley
- 6 cups reduced-sodium chicken broth
- 2 cups cooked turkey breast, cubed
- 2 cups fresh baby spinach
- ½ teaspoon pepper

Preparation:
1. Add the oil to a saucepan, then heat it over medium-high.
2. Stir in the onion and carrots to sauté for 5 minutes.
3. Add the broth and barley and bring to a boil.
4. Reduce the heat to a low simmer. Cook for 15 minutes.
5. Stir in the pepper, spinach, and turkey.
6. Mix well and serve.

Serving Suggestion: Serve the soup with fresh bread.
Variation Tip: Add shredded cheese on top.
Nutritional Information per Serving:
Calories 208 | Fat 12g |Sodium 70mg | Carbs 23g | Fiber 6g | Sugar 3g | Protein 21g

Hasselback Eggplant Parmesan

Prep Time: 1 hour 20 minutes
Cook Time: 25 minutes
Serves: 4
Ingredients:

- 1 cup prepared low-sodium marinara sauce
- 4 small eggplants (about 6 inches long; 1¾ lbs. total)
- 2 tbsp. extra-virgin olive oil plus 2 tsp., divided
- 4 oz. fresh mozzarella, thinly sliced into 12 pieces
- ¼ cup prepared pesto
- ½ cup whole-wheat panko breadcrumbs
- 2 tbsp. grated parmesan cheese
- 1 tbsp. chopped fresh basil

Preparation:
1. Preheat the oven to 375°F.
2. Spread the marinara sauce in a 9 x 13-inch broiler-safe baking dish.
3. Make crosswise cuts every ¼ inch along each eggplant, slicing almost to the bottom but not all the way through.
4. Carefully transfer the eggplants to the baking dish. Gently fan them to open the cuts wider. Drizzle 2 tbsp. of oil over the eggplants. Fill the cuts alternately with mozzarella and pesto (some cuts may not be filled). Cover with foil.
5. Bake until the eggplants are very tender, 45 to 55 minutes.
6. Combine the panko, parmesan, and the remaining oil in a small bowl. Remove the foil and sprinkle the eggplants with the breadcrumb mixture.
7. Change the oven setting to broil. Broil the eggplants on the center rack until the topping is golden brown, 2 to 4 minutes. Top with the basil.

Serving Suggestion: Serve the eggplant with the sauce.
Variation Tip: Add different spices of your choice.
Nutritional Information Per Serving:
Calories 349 | Protein 14.4g | Carbohydrates 24.3g | Dietary fiber 7.3g | Sugars 9.4g | Fat 22.8g | Sodium 405.1mg

Walnut-Rosemary Crusted Salmon

Prep Time: 20 minutes
Cook Time: 10 minutes
Serves: 4
Ingredients
- 2 tsp. Dijon mustard
- 1 clove garlic, minced
- ¼ tsp. lemon zest
- 1 tsp. lemon juice
- 1 tsp. chopped fresh rosemary

- ½ tsp. honey
- ½ tsp. kosher salt
- ¼ tsp. crushed red pepper
- 3 tbsp. panko breadcrumbs
- 3 tbsp. finely chopped walnuts
- 1 tsp. extra-virgin olive oil
- 1 (1 lb.) skinless salmon fillet, fresh or frozen
- Olive oil cooking spray
- Chopped fresh parsley and lemon wedges for garnish

Preparation

1. Preheat the oven to 425°F. Line a large rimmed baking sheet with parchment paper.
2. Combine the mustard, garlic, lemon zest, lemon juice, rosemary, honey, salt, and crushed red pepper in a small bowl.
3. Combine the panko, walnuts, and oil in another small bowl.
4. Place the salmon on the prepared baking sheet. Spread the mustard mixture over the fish and sprinkle with the panko mixture, pressing to adhere. Lightly coat with cooking spray.
5. Bake until the fish flakes easily with a fork, about 8 to 12 minutes, depending on thickness.

Serving Suggestion: Serve with a tortilla.

Variation Tip: Sprinkle with parsley and serve with lemon wedges, if desired.

Nutritional Information Per Serving:
Calories 222 | Protein 24g | Carbohydrates 4g | Dietary fiber 2g | Sugars 1g | Fat 12g | Sodium 256mg

Chicken Caesar Pasta Salad

Prep Time: 30 minutes
Cook Time: 20 minutes
Serves: 6
Ingredients
- ½ cup low-fat buttermilk
- ¼ cup low-fat plain Greek yogurt
- 3 tbsp. extra-virgin olive oil
- 2 tbsp. fresh lemon juice
- 2 tsp. Dijon mustard
- 1½ tsp. anchovy paste
- 1 large garlic clove
- ¾ cup finely grated parmesan cheese, divided
- ½ tsp. salt, divided
- ½ tsp. ground pepper, divided
- 8 oz. whole-wheat penne
- 3 cups shredded cooked chicken breast
- 1 pint cherry tomatoes, halved
- 5 cups chopped romaine lettuce

Preparation

1. Combine the buttermilk, yogurt, oil, lemon juice, mustard, anchovy paste, garlic, ½ cup parmesan, and ¼ tsp. each of salt and pepper in a blender. Puree on high speed until smooth, about 1 minute. Set aside.
2. Cook the pasta according to package directions, omitting salt. Drain, reserving 1 cup of the cooking water.
3. Combine the pasta, chicken, tomatoes, ¼ cup of the reserved cooking water, and the remaining ¼ tsp. each of salt and pepper in a large bowl.
4. Stir in the buttermilk dressing until thoroughly combined. Stir in the additional cooking water as needed for a creamy consistency.
5. Cover and chill for at least 30 minutes or up to 2 days.

Serving Suggestion: Just before serving, stir in the lettuce and sprinkle with the remaining ¼ cup parmesan.

Variation Tip: Add dried herbs or spices of your choice for added flavor.

Nutritional Information Per Serving:
Calories 383 | Protein 32.8g | Carbohydrates 33.8g | Dietary fiber 4.4g | Sugars 4g | Fat 13.6g | Sodium 571.8mg

Eating Well Eggplant Parmesan

Prep Time: 45 minutes
Cook Time: 25 minutes
Serves: 6
Ingredients
- Canola or olive oil cooking spray
- 2 large eggs
- 2 tbsp. water
- 1 cup panko breadcrumbs
- ¾ cup grated parmesan cheese, divided
- 1 tsp. Italian seasoning
- 2 medium eggplants (about 2 lbs. total), cut crosswise into ¼-inch-thick slices
- ½ tsp. salt
- ½ tsp. ground pepper
- 1 (24 oz.) jar no-salt-added tomato sauce
- ¼ cup fresh basil leaves, torn, plus more for serving
- 2 cloves garlic, grated
- ½ tsp. crushed red pepper
- 1 cup shredded part-skim mozzarella cheese, divided

Preparation

1. Position racks in the middle and lower thirds of the oven. Preheat to 400°F. Coat two baking sheets and a 9 x 13-inch baking dish with cooking spray.
2. Whisk the eggs and water in a shallow bowl.
3. Mix the breadcrumbs, ¼ cup parmesan, and Italian seasoning in another shallow dish.

4. Dip the eggplant in the egg mixture, then coat with the breadcrumb mixture, gently pressing to adhere.
5. Arrange the eggplant in a single layer on the prepared baking sheets. Generously spray both sides of the eggplant with cooking spray. Bake, flipping the eggplant, and switching the pans between racks halfway until the eggplant is tender and lightly browned, about 30 minutes. Season with salt and pepper.
6. Meanwhile, mix the tomato sauce, basil, garlic, and crushed red pepper in a medium bowl.
7. Spread about ½ cup of the sauce in a prepared baking dish. Arrange half the eggplant slices over the sauce. Spoon 1 cup sauce over the eggplant and sprinkle with ¼ cup parmesan and ½ cup mozzarella. Top with the remaining eggplant, sauce, and cheese.
8. Bake until the sauce is bubbling and the top is golden, 20 to 30 minutes. Let cool for 5 minutes. Sprinkle with more basil before serving, if desired.
Serving Suggestion: Serve with tortilla or bread.
Variation Tip: Sprinkle with more basil before serving, if desired.
Nutritional Information Per Serving:
Calories 241 | Protein 14g | Carbohydrates 28g | Dietary fiber 6g| Sugars 9g | Fat 9g | Sodium 553mg

Mediterranean Chicken Quinoa Bowl

Prep Time: 30 minutes
Cook Time: 30 minutes
Serves: 4
Ingredients
- 1 lb. boneless, skinless chicken breasts, trimmed
- ¼ tsp. salt
- ¼ tsp. ground pepper
- 1 (7 oz.) jar roasted red peppers, rinsed
- ¼ cup slivered almonds
- 4 tbsp. extra-virgin olive oil, divided
- 1 small clove garlic, crushed
- 1 tsp. paprika
- ½ tsp. ground cumin
- ¼ tsp. crushed red pepper (optional)
- 2 cups cooked quinoa
- ¼ cup pitted Kalamata olives, chopped
- ¼ cup finely chopped red onion
- 1 cup diced cucumber
- ¼ cup crumbled feta cheese
- 2 tbsp. finely chopped fresh parsley
Preparation

1. Position a rack in the upper third of the oven. Preheat the broiler to high. Line a rimmed baking sheet with foil.
2. Sprinkle the chicken with the salt and pepper and place it on the prepared baking sheet.
3. Broil the chicken, turning it once, until an instant-read thermometer inserted in the thickest part reads 165°F (about 14 to 18 minutes). Transfer the chicken to a clean cutting board and slice or shred.
4. Meanwhile, place the peppers, almonds, 2 tbsp. of oil, the garlic, paprika, cumin, and crushed red pepper (if using) in a mini food processor. Puree until fairly smooth.
5. Combine the quinoa, olives, red onion, and the remaining oil in a medium bowl.
Serving Suggestion: Divide the quinoa mixture among four bowls and top with equal amounts of cucumber, chicken, and red pepper sauce. Sprinkle with the feta and parsley.
Variation Tip: Prepare the chicken (Steps 2 to 3), red pepper sauce (Step 3), and quinoa (Step 4). Refrigerate in separate containers. Assemble just before serving.
Nutritional Information Per Serving:
Calories 519 | Protein 34.1g | Carbohydrates 31.2g | Dietary fiber 4.2g | Sugars 2.5g | Fat 26.9g | Sodium 683.5mg

Chicken and Vegetable Penne with Parsley-Walnut Pesto

Prep Time: 30 minutes
Cook Time: 20 minutes
Serves: 4
Ingredients
- ¾ cup chopped walnuts
- 1 cup lightly packed parsley leaves
- 2 cloves garlic, crushed and peeled
- ½ tsp. salt (plus ⅛ tsp.)
- ⅛ tsp. ground pepper
- 2 tbsp. olive oil
- ⅓ cup grated parmesan cheese
- 1½ cups shredded or sliced cooked skinless chicken breast (8 oz.)
- 6 oz. whole-wheat penne or fusilli pasta (1¾ cups)
- 2 cups green beans, trimmed and halved crosswise
- 2 cups cauliflower florets
Preparation
1. Bring a large pot of water to a boil.

2. Place the walnuts in a small bowl and microwave on high until fragrant and lightly toasted, 2 to 2½ minutes. (Alternatively, toast the walnuts in a small dry skillet over medium-low heat, stirring constantly, until fragrant, 2 to 3 minutes.) Transfer to a plate and let cool. Set ¼ cup aside for topping.

3. In a food processor, combine the remaining ½ cup walnuts, parsley, garlic, salt, and pepper. Process until the nuts are ground. With the motor running, gradually add oil through the feed tube. Add the parmesan and pulse until mixed in. Scrape the pesto into a large bowl. Add the chicken.

4. Meanwhile, cook the pasta in the boiling water for 4 minutes. Add the green beans and cauliflower. Cover and cook until the pasta is al dente (almost tender) and the vegetables are tender, 5 to 7 minutes more. Before draining, scoop out ¾ cup of the cooking water and stir it into the pesto-chicken mixture to warm it slightly. Drain the pasta and vegetables and add to the pesto-chicken mixture. Toss to coat well.

Serving Suggestion: Divide among four pasta bowls and top each serving with 1 tbsp. of the reserved walnuts.

Variation Tip: Add spices of your choice.

Nutritional Information Per Serving:
Calories 514 | Protein 31.4g | Carbohydrates 43.4g | Dietary fiber 8.6g | Sugars 4.8g | Fat 26.6g | Sodium 556.6mg

Greek Chicken With Roasted Spring Vegetables and Lemon Vinaigrette

Prep Time: 50 minutes
Cook Time: 30 minutes
Serves: 4
Ingredients
Lemon Vinaigrette:
• 1 lemon
• 1 tbsp. olive oil
• 1 tbsp. crumbled feta cheese
• ½ tsp. honey
Greek Chicken and Vegetables:
• 2 (8 oz.) skinless, boneless chicken breast halves, cut in half lengthwise
• ¼ cup light mayonnaise
• 6 cloves garlic, minced
• ½ cup panko breadcrumbs
• 3 tbsp. grated parmesan cheese
• ½ tsp. kosher salt
• ½ tsp. black pepper
• Non-stick olive oil cooking spray
• 2 cups 1-inch pieces asparagus

• 1½ cups sliced fresh cremini mushrooms
• 1½ cups halved grape tomatoes
• 1 tbsp. olive oil
• Snipped fresh dill
Preparation
1. To prepare the vinaigrette: Remove ½ tsp. of zest and squeeze 1 tbsp. of juice from the lemon. In a small bowl, whisk together the lemon zest and juice and the remaining ingredients. Set aside.

2. To prepare the chicken and vegetables: Preheat oven to 475°F. Place a 15 x 10-inch baking pan into the oven.

3. Meanwhile, using the flat side of a meat mallet, flatten the chicken between two pieces of plastic wrap until ½ inch thick.

4. Place the chicken in a medium bowl. Add the mayonnaise and 2 of the garlic cloves. Stir to coat.

5. In a shallow dish, stir together the breadcrumbs, cheese, ¼ tsp. of the salt, and ¼ tsp. of the pepper.

6. Dip the chicken into the crumb mixture, turning to coat. Lightly coat the tops of the chicken with cooking spray.

7. In a large bowl, combine the asparagus, mushrooms, tomatoes, oil, and the remaining 4 cloves of garlic and ¼ tsp. of salt and pepper.

8. Carefully place the chicken on one end of the hot pan and place the asparagus mixture on the other end. Roast for 18 to 20 minutes or until the chicken is done (165°F) and the vegetables are tender.

Serving Suggestion: Drizzle the chicken and vegetables with the vinaigrette and sprinkle with dill.

Variation Tip: Add spices of your choice.

Nutritional Information Per Serving:
Calories 306 | Protein 29.5g | Carbohydrates 12.1g | Dietary fiber 1.6g | Sugars 3.6g | Fat 15.1g | Sodium 431.5mg

Thai Chicken Pasta

Prep Time: 10 minutes
Cook Time: 15 minutes
Serves: 4
Ingredients:
• 6 ounces whole-wheat spaghetti
• 2 teaspoons canola oil
• 10 ounces snap peas, sliced
• 2 cups carrots, julienned
• 2 cups cooked chicken, shredded
• 1 cup Thai peanut sauce
• 1 medium cucumber, sliced
• Chopped fresh cilantro, optional
Preparation:
1. Boil and cook the spaghetti as per the given instructions on the packet. Drain and rinse under cold water.

2. Heat a skillet greased with oil on medium heat.

3. Add the carrots and snap peas. Sauté for 8 minutes.

4. Stir in the peanut sauce, chicken and spaghetti.
5. Toss well and cook until well mixed.
6. Garnish with cilantro and cucumber.
7. Serve.
Serving Suggestion: Serve the meal with a bowl of Greek salad.
Variation Tip: Add a drop of hot sauce for a spicy flavor.
Nutritional Information per Serving:
Calories 409 | Fat 5g |Sodium 50mg | Carbs 43g | Fiber 5g | Sugar 4g | Protein 21g

Dijon Salmon With Green Bean Pilaf

Prep Time: 30 minutes
Cook Time: 10 minutes
Serves: 4
Ingredients
• 1¼ lbs. wild salmon, skinned and cut into 4 portions
• 3 tbsp. extra-virgin olive oil, divided
• 1 tbsp. minced garlic
• ¾ tsp. salt
• 2 tbsp. mayonnaise
• 2 tsp. whole-grain mustard
• ½ tsp. ground pepper, divided
• 12 oz. pretrimmed haricots verts or thin green beans, cut into thirds
• 1 small lemon, zested and cut into 4 wedges
• 2 tbsp. pine nuts
• 8 oz. precooked brown rice
• 2 tbsp. water
• Chopped fresh parsley for garnish
Preparation
1. Preheat the oven to 425°F. Line a rimmed baking sheet with foil or parchment paper.
2. Brush the salmon with 1 tbsp. of oil and place on the prepared baking sheet.
3. Mash the garlic and salt into a paste with the side of a chef's knife or a fork. Combine a scant 1 tsp. of the garlic paste in a small bowl with mayonnaise, mustard, and ¼ tsp. of pepper. Spread the mixture on top of the fish.
4. Roast the salmon until it flakes easily with a fork in the thickest part, 6 to 8 minutes per inch of thickness.
5. Meanwhile, heat the remaining 2 tbsp. of oil in a large skillet over medium-high heat. Add the green beans, lemon zest, pine nuts, the remaining garlic paste, and ¼ tsp. of pepper. Cook, stirring, until the beans are just tender, 2 to 4 minutes.
6. Reduce the heat to medium. Add the rice and water and cook, stirring, until hot, 2 to 3 minutes more.

Serving Suggestion: Sprinkle the salmon with parsley, if desired, and serve with the green bean pilaf and lemon wedges.
Variation Tip: Add spices or herbs of your choice.
Nutritional Information Per Serving:
Calories 442 | Protein 32.2g | Carbohydrates 21.6g | Dietary fiber 3.8g | Sugars 1.7g | Fat 24.8g | Sodium 605.2mg

Chicken Souvlaki Kabobs With Mediterranean Couscous

Prep Time: 2 hours 20 minutes
Cook Time: 45 minutes
Serves: 4
Ingredients

Chicken Souvlaki Kabobs:
• 1 lb. skinless, boneless chicken breast halves, cut into ½-inch strips
• 1 cup sliced fennel (reserve the leaves, if desired)
• ⅓ cup dry white wine
• ¼ cup lemon juice
• 3 tbsp. canola oil
• 4 cloves garlic, minced
• 2 tsp. dried oregano, crushed
• ½ tsp. salt
• ¼ tsp. black pepper
• Lemon wedges
Mediterranean Couscous:
• 1 tsp. olive oil
• ½ cup Israeli (large pearl) couscous
• 1 cup water
• ½ cup snipped dried tomatoes (not oil-packed)
• ¾ cup chopped red sweet pepper
• ½ cup chopped cucumber
• ½ cup chopped red onion
• ⅓ cup plain fat-free Greek yogurt
• ¼ cup thinly sliced fresh basil leaves
• ¼ cup snipped fresh parsley
• 1 tbsp. lemon juice
• ¼ tsp. salt
• ¼ tsp. black pepper
Preparation
1. To prepare the kabobs: Place the chicken and sliced fennel in a resealable plastic bag and set the bag in a shallow dish. Combine the white wine, lemon juice, oil, garlic, oregano, salt, and pepper in a small bowl for the marinade. Remove ¼ cup of the marinade and set aside.

2. Pour the remaining marinade over the chicken mixture. Seal the bag and turn it over to coat the chicken mixture. Marinate in the refrigerator for 1½ hours, turning the bag once.

3. Meanwhile, prepare your skewers. If using wooden skewers, soak eight 10- to 12-inch skewers in water for 30 minutes. Drain the chicken, discarding the marinade and the fennel. Thread the chicken, accordion-style, onto the skewers.

4. Grill the chicken skewers, covered, over medium-high heat for 6 to 8 minutes or until the chicken is no longer pink, turning once. Remove from the grill and brush with the reserved ¼ cup marinade.

5. To prepare the couscous: In a small saucepan, heat 1 tsp. of olive oil over medium heat. Add ½ cup Israeli (large pearl) couscous. Cook and stir for 4 minutes or until light brown. Add 1 cup water. Bring to a boil and then reduce the heat. Simmer, covered, for 10 minutes or until the couscous is tender and the liquid is absorbed. Add ½ cup of snipped dried tomatoes (not oil-packed) in the last 5 minutes.

6. Cool the couscous and then transfer it to a large bowl. Stir in ¾ cup chopped red sweet pepper, ½ cup each chopped cucumber and chopped red onion, ⅓ cup plain fat-free Greek yogurt, ¼ cup each thinly sliced fresh basil leaves, snipped fresh parsley, 1 tbsp. lemon juice, and ¼ tsp. each of salt and black pepper.

Serving Suggestion: Serve with tortillas.

Variation Tip: Serve the kabobs with couscous, lemon wedges, and, if desired, the reserved fennel leaves.

Nutritional Information Per Serving:
Calories 332 | Protein 32.1g | Carbohydrates 27.7g | Dietary fiber 2.3g | Sugars 6.4g | Fat 9.4g| Sodium 360mg.

Chicken and Spring Vegetable Tortellini Salad

Prep Time: 30 minutes
Cook Time: 30 minutes
Serves: 6
Ingredients
- 1 lb. boneless, skinless chicken breast
- 2 bay leaves
- 6 cups water
- 1 (20 oz.) package fresh cheese tortellini
- ½ cup peas, fresh or frozen
- ¼ cup creamy salad dressing, such as ranch or peppercorn

- 2 tbsp. red-wine vinegar
- 5 tbsp. chopped fresh herbs, such as basil, dill, and/or chives, divided
- ½ cup chopped marinated artichokes plus 2 tbsp. marinade, divided
- ½ cup julienned radishes
- 1 cup pea shoots or baby arugula
- 2 tbsp. sunflower seeds

Preparation
1. Combine the chicken, bay leaves, and water in a large saucepan. Bring to a boil over high heat. Reduce the heat to low, cover, and simmer until an instant-read thermometer inserted in the thickest part registers 165°F (around 10 to 12 minutes). Transfer the chicken to a clean cutting board to cool.

2. Remove the bay leaves. Add the tortellini to the pot and return the water to a boil. Cook, stirring occasionally, until the tortellini are just tender, about 3 minutes.

3. Add the peas and cook for 1 minute more. Drain and rinse with cold water.

4. Meanwhile, combine the dressing, vinegar, 3 tbsp. of the fresh herbs, and the artichoke marinade in a large bowl.

5. Shred the chicken and add to the dressing along with the tortellini, peas, artichokes, radishes, and pea shoots (or arugula). Stir to combine.

Serving Suggestion: Serve the salad topped with the remaining 2 tbsp. of the herbs and the sunflower seeds.

Variation Tip: Add vegetables of your choice.

Nutritional Information Per Serving:
Calories 357 | Protein 23.6g | Carbohydrates 35.5g | Dietary fiber 3.8g | Sugars 2.9g | Fat 12.7g | Sodium 452.1mg

Creamy Lemon Pasta with Shrimp

Prep Time: 20 minutes
Cook Time: 20 minutes
Serves: 4
Ingredients
- 8 oz. whole-wheat fettuccine
- 1 tbsp. extra-virgin olive oil
- 12 oz. sustainably sourced, peeled, and deveined raw shrimp (26–30 per lb.)
- 2 tbsp. unsalted butter
- 1 tbsp. finely chopped garlic
- ¼ tsp. crushed red pepper
- 4 cups loosely packed arugula
- ¼ cup whole-milk plain yogurt
- 1 tsp. lemon zest

- 2 tbsp. lemon juice
- ¼ tsp. salt
- ⅓ cup grated parmesan cheese, plus more for garnish
- ¼ cup thinly sliced fresh basil

Preparation

1. Bring 7 cups of water to a boil. Add the fettuccine, stirring to separate the noodles. Cook until just tender, 7 to 9 minutes. Reserve ½ cup of the cooking water and drain.
2. Meanwhile, heat the oil in a large non-stick skillet over medium-high heat. Add the shrimp and cook, stirring occasionally, until pink and curled, 2 to 3 minutes. Transfer the shrimp to a bowl.
3. Add the butter to the pan and reduce the heat to medium. Add the garlic and crushed red pepper. Cook, stirring often, until the garlic is fragrant, about 1 minute.
4. Add the arugula and cook, stirring, until wilted, about 1 minute. Reduce the heat to low.
5. Add the fettuccine, yogurt, lemon zest, and the reserved cooking water, ¼ cup at a time, tossing well, until the fettuccine is fully coated and creamy.
6. Add the shrimp, lemon juice, and salt, tossing to coat the fettuccine. Remove from the heat and toss with parmesan.

Serving Suggestion: Serve with tortillas.
Variation Tip: Serve the fettuccine topped with basil and more parmesan, if desired.
Nutritional Information Per Serving:
Calories 403 | Protein 28.3g | Carbohydrates 45.5g | Dietary fiber 5.8g | Sugars 3g | Fat 13.9g | Sodium 396.3mg

Mediterranean Chickpea Quinoa Bowl

Prep Time: 20 minutes
Cook Time: 20 minutes
Serves: 4
Ingredients
- 1 (7 oz.) jar roasted red peppers, rinsed
- ¼ cup slivered almonds
- 4 tbsp. extra-virgin olive oil, divided
- 1 small clove garlic, minced
- 1 tsp. paprika
- ½ tsp. ground cumin
- ¼ tsp. crushed red pepper (optional)
- 2 cups cooked quinoa
- ¼ cup Kalamata olives, chopped
- ¼ cup finely chopped red onion
- 1 (15 oz.) can chickpeas, rinsed

- 1 cup diced cucumber
- ¼ cup crumbled feta cheese
- 2 tbsp. finely chopped fresh parsley

Preparation

1. Place the peppers, almonds, 2 tbsp. of oil, garlic, paprika, cumin, and crushed red pepper (if using) in a mini food processor. Puree until fairly smooth.
2. Combine the quinoa, olives, red onion, and the remaining 2 tbsp. of oil in a medium bowl.

Serving Suggestion: Divide the quinoa mixture among four bowls. Top with equal amounts of chickpeas, cucumber, and red pepper sauce. Sprinkle with feta and parsley.
Variation Tip: To make ahead: Prepare the red pepper sauce (Step 1) and quinoa (Step 2). Refrigerate in separate containers. Assemble just before serving.
Nutritional Information Per Serving:
Calories 479 | Protein 12.7g | Carbohydrates 49.5g | Dietary fiber 7.7g | Sugars 2.5g | Fat 24.8g | Sodium 646mg

Cherry Chicken Wraps

Prep Time: 10 minutes
Cook Time: 10 minutes
Serves: 8
Ingredients:
- ¾ pound boneless chicken breasts, cut into cubes
- 1 teaspoon ground ginger
- ¼ teaspoon salt
- ¼ teaspoon pepper
- 2 teaspoons olive oil
- 1½ cups shredded carrots
- 1¼ cups pitted fresh sweet cherries, chopped
- 4 green onions, chopped
- ⅓ cup almonds, coarsely chopped
- 2 tablespoons rice vinegar
- 2 tablespoons low sodium teriyaki sauce
- 1 tablespoon honey
- 8 Boston lettuce leaves
- 8 tortilla wraps

Preparation:

1. Season the chicken with the salt, pepper, and ginger.
2. Heat a skillet greased with oil on medium heat.
3. Add the chicken and cook for 5 minutes until it changes its color.
4. Stir in the cherries, almonds, green onions, and carrots.
5. Add the honey, teriyaki, and vinegar. Mix well.
6. Spread the tortilla with lettuce leaves on top on a serving plate.

7. Spread the chicken mixture over the lettuce.

8. Fold the wraps and serve.

Serving Suggestion: Serve the meal with a bowl of broccoli salad.

Variation Tip: Add shredded cabbage to the filling.

Nutritional Information per Serving:

Calories 257 | Fat 7g |Sodium 69mg | Carbs 25g | Fiber 4g | Sugar 12g | Protein 21g

Fajita Chili

Prep Time: 15 minutes

Cook Time: 5 hours

Serves: 8

Ingredients:

- 2 pounds boneless chicken breast, cut into 1-inch chunks
- 1 tablespoon chili powder
- 1 teaspoon fajita seasoning
- ½ teaspoon ground cumin
- 2 garlic cloves, minced
- Non-stick cooking spray
- 2 x 14½-ounce cans diced tomatoes
- ½ green bell pepper, julienned
- ½ red bell pepper, julienned
- ½ yellow bell pepper, julienned
- ½ onion, sliced
- 1 x 15-ounce can white kidney beans, rinsed and drained
- 3 tablespoons sour cream
- 3 tablespoons reduced-fat cheddar cheese, shredded
- 3 tablespoons guacamole

Preparation:

1. Mix the chicken with the cumin, garlic, fajita seasoning, and chili powder in a bowl.

2. Heat a skillet greased with cooking spray on medium heat.

3. Add the chicken and sauté until golden brown.

4. Transfer the chicken to a slow cooker.

5. Add the vegetables, undrained tomatoes, and cannellini beans to the slow cooker.

6. Cover and cook on a low setting for 5 hours.

7. Garnish with sour cream, guacamole, and shredded cheese.

8. Serve.

Serving Suggestion: Serve the chili with a bowl of spinach salad.

Variation Tip: Add some smoked paprika for seasoning.

Nutritional Information per Serving:

Calories 225 | Fat 16g |Sodium 55mg | Carbs 21g | Fiber 1.2g | Sugar 5g | Protein 21g

Vegetable Polenta

Prep Time: 10 minutes

Cook Time: 20 minutes

Serves: 6

Ingredients:

- 1 eggplant, peeled, cut into slices
- 1 yellow zucchini, cut into slices
- 1 green zucchini, cut into slices
- 6 mushrooms, sliced
- 1 cored sweet red pepper, chopped
- 2½ tablespoons olive oil
- 6 cups water
- 1½ cups coarse polenta
- 2 teaspoons margarine
- ¼ teaspoon cracked black pepper
- 10 ounces frozen spinach, thawed
- 2 plum (Roma) tomatoes, sliced
- 6 dry-packed sun-dried tomatoes, drained and chopped
- 10 ripe olives, chopped
- 2 teaspoons oregano

Preparation:

1. Preheat the broiler and set its rack 4 inches below the heat source.

2. Toss the eggplant, mushrooms, red pepper, and zucchini with 1 tablespoon of the oil.

3. Add the veggies to a baking sheet and broil, flipping them every few minutes.

4. Brush the veggies with more oil if needed and cook until they turn brown.

5. Preheat the oven to 350°F.

6. Layer a 12-inch quiche pan with cooking spray.

7. Boil the water with the polenta in a saucepan, then reduce the heat to a simmer.

8. Cook the polenta for 5 minutes, then add the margarine and black pepper to taste.

9. Spread the cooked polenta in the quiche pan and top it with the spinach, tomatoes, sun-dried tomatoes, and olives.
10. Add the remaining roasted vegetables on top.
11. Sprinkle the oregano and black pepper over it.
12. Bake for 10 minutes, then slice.
13. Serve.
Serving Suggestion: Serve the meal with a bowl of cucumber salad.
Variation Tip: Add chopped tomatoes on top.
Nutritional Information per Serving:
Calories 215 | Fat 9.4g |Sodium 189mg | Carbs 23g | Fiber 0.3g | Sugar 18.2g | Protein 37g

Linguini Chicken Soup

Prep Time: 10 minutes
Cook Time: 20 minutes
Serves: 6
Ingredients:
• 1 teaspoon olive oil
• 1 cup onion, chopped
• 3 garlic cloves, minced
• 1 cup celery, chopped
• 1 cup carrots, sliced and peeled
• 4 cups chicken broth
• 4 ounces dried linguini, broken
• 1 cup cooked chicken breast, cut into the desired size
• 2 tablespoons fresh parsley
Preparation:
1. Add the olive oil to a saucepan, then heat it on medium flame.
2. Stir in the garlic and onion. Sauté until soft.
3. Add the carrots and celery. Stir and cook for 3 minutes.
4. Pour in the broth and cook until it boils, then reduce it to a simmer.
5. Cook for 5 minutes, then add the linguini.
6. Bring to a boil and then reduce the heat to a simmer.
7. Cook for 10 more minutes.
8. Add the chicken and parsley.
9. Cook for a minute, then serve warm.
Serving Suggestion: Serve with fresh bread.
Variation Tip: Add peas or chopped mushrooms to the soup.
Nutritional Information per Serving:
Calories 381 | Fat 15g |Sodium 42mg | Carbs 9.7g | Fiber 0.4g | Sugar 1g | Protein 25.2g

Fajita Chicken Wraps

Prep Time: 10 minutes
Cook Time: 6 minutes
Serves: 2
Ingredients:
• 12 ounces skinless chicken breast strips
• ½ teaspoon chili powder
• ¼ teaspoon garlic powder
• Non-stick cooking spray
• 1 red or green sweet pepper, seeded and cut into strips
• 2 tablespoons bottled ranch salad dressing
• 2 x 10-inch whole-wheat tortillas
• ½ cup salsa
• ⅓ cup reduced-fat cheddar cheese, shredded
Preparation:
1. Mix the chicken strips with the garlic powder and chili powder.
2. Heat a skillet greased with cooking spray on medium heat.
3. Add the chicken and sweet peppers. Cook for 6 minutes.
4. Toss in the ranch salad dressing.
5. Divide the mixture into warmed tortillas.
6. Top each tortilla with cheese and salsa.
7. Roll each tortilla and cut them in half.
8. Serve.
Serving Suggestion: Serve the meal with a bowl of kale salad.
Variation Tip: Add coleslaw to the wraps.
Nutritional Information per Serving:
Calories 245 | Fat 17g |Sodium 42mg | Carbs 8.7g | Fiber 0g | Sugar 1g | Protein 38.5g

Black Bean Cheese Wrap

Prep Time: 10 minutes
Cook Time: 2 minutes
Serves: 6
Ingredients:
• 1½ cups black beans, drained

- 3 tablespoons cilantro, chopped
- 1½ cups corn kernels
- 2 tablespoons green chili peppers, chopped
- 4 green onions, diced
- 1 tomato, diced
- 1 tablespoon chopped garlic
- 6 fat-free whole-grain tortilla wraps
- ¾ cup shredded cheddar cheese
- ¾ cup salsa

Preparation:
1. Toss the black beans with the corn, chili peppers, onions, garlic, tomato, and cilantro in a bowl.
2. Heat the mixture in a microwave for 1 minute, stirring halfway through.
3. Spread 2 tortillas between paper towels and heat them in the microwave for 20 secs.
4. Warm the remaining tortillas in the same way.
5. Add ½ cup of the bean mixture, 2 tablespoons of salsa, and 2 tablespoons of cheese to each tortilla.
6. Roll them and serve instantly.

Serving Suggestion: Serve the wraps with a bowl of spinach salad.

Variation Tip: Add shredded cabbage to the wrap.

Nutritional Information per Serving:
Calories 280 | Fat 8g |Sodium 39mg | Carbs 26g |
Fiber 1g | Sugar 2g | Protein 12g

Garlic Beef Brisket

Prep Time: 10 minutes
Cook Time: 3 hours and 10 minutes
Serves: 4
Ingredients:
- 1 tablespoon olive oil
- 2½ pounds beef brisket, cut into pieces
- Ground black pepper, to taste
- 1½ cups onions, chopped
- 4 garlic cloves, smashed and peeled
- 1 teaspoon dried thyme
- 1 can (14½ ounces) tomatoes (with its liquid)
- ¼ cup red wine vinegar
- 1 cup low-sodium beef stock

Preparation:
1. Preheat the oven to 350°F.
2. Grease a Dutch oven with 1 tablespoon of oil and heat on a medium flame.
3. Add the ground pepper to the brisket for seasoning and sauté in the Dutch oven until it turns brown.
4. Transfer the seared brisket to a plate.
5. Add the onions to the same pot and sauté until golden brown.
6. Stir in the thyme and garlic and cook for 1 minute.
7. Add the vinegar, stock, and tomatoes.
8. Bring the mixture to a boil and return the brisket to the pot.

9. Reduce the heat to a simmer and cook for 3 hours or more until the meat is tender.
10. Serve warm.

Serving Suggestion: Serve the meal with a bowl of tomato and cucumber salad.

Variation Tip: You can add chopped carrots to the brisket as well.

Nutritional Information per Serving:
Calories 209 | Fat 9g |Sodium 72mg | Carbs 21.4g |
Fiber 1.3g | Sugar 1.2g | Protein 10.2g

Beef Fennel Stew

Prep Time: 25 minutes
Cook Time: 1 hour and 30 minutes
Serves: 4
Ingredients:
- 3 tablespoons all-purpose flour
- 1 pound lean boneless beef, cut into cubes
- 2 tablespoons olive oil
- ½ fennel bulb, sliced vertically
- 3 large shallots, chopped
- ¾ teaspoon ground black pepper
- 2 fresh thyme sprigs
- 1 bay leaf
- 3 cups vegetable stock
- ½ cup red wine, optional
- 4 carrots, peeled and cut into 1-inch pieces
- 4 large white potatoes, peeled and cubed
- 18 small boiling onions, halved crosswise
- 3 portobello mushrooms, diced
- ⅓ cup fresh flat-leaf parsley, chopped

Preparation:
1. Spread the flour in a shallow container or plate.
2. Add the beef cubes and dredge them in the flour to coat well, then shake off the excess.
3. Take a large saucepan and add the oil to it. Heat over medium flame.
4. Add the beef and sauté for 5 minutes, then transfer it to a plate using a slotted spoon.
5. Add the shallots and fennel to the same saucepan and sauté for 7 minutes.
6. Stir in the thyme, bay leaf, and pepper. Cook for 1 minute.
7. Add the beef to the pan along with the wine and stock.
8. Bring to a boil and then reduce it to a simmer. Cover it and cook for 45 minutes.
9. Now add the mushrooms, onions, potatoes, and carrots.
10. Cook for 30 minutes until the vegetables are soft.
11. Remove the bay leaf and thyme sprigs.
12. Garnish with parsley.
13. Serve warm.

Serving Suggestion: Serve the meal with a bowl of Greek salad.

Variation Tip: Add paprika and dried herbs to season the stew.

Nutritional Information per Serving:
Calories 384 | Fat 2g |Sodium 60mg | Carbs 26g | Fiber 0.4g | Sugar 2g | Protein 32g

Tuscan Croutons Bean Stew

Prep Time: 15 minutes
Cook Time: 1 hour and 30 minutes
Serves: 6
Ingredients:
Croutons:
- 1 tablespoon olive oil
- 2 garlic cloves, quartered
- 1 slice whole-grain bread, cut into ½-inch cubes

Soup:
- 2 cups white beans, soaked and drained
- 6 cups water
- 1 bay leaf
- 2 tablespoons olive oil
- 1 cup yellow onion, chopped
- 3 carrots, peeled and chopped
- 6 garlic cloves, chopped
- ¼ teaspoon black pepper
- 1 tablespoon fresh rosemary chopped
- 1½ cups low-sodium vegetable stock

Preparation:
1. Add the oil to a large skillet and heat it.
2. Stir in the garlic and sauté for 1 minute.
3. Let it sit for 10 minutes, then remove the garlic from the oil.
4. Return the skillet with the oil to the heat and add the bread cubes.
5. Sauté for 5 minutes until golden brown, then set them aside.
6. Mix the white beans, water, and bay leaf in a pot.
7. Boil the beans on high heat, then reduce the heat to a simmer.
8. Partially cover the beans, then cook for 60 to 70 minutes until al dente.
9. Drain the beans and keep a ½ cup of the cooking liquid.
10. Discard the bay leaf and transfer the beans to a bowl.
11. Mix the reserved liquid with ½ cup of the beans in a bowl.
12. Mash this mixture to form a paste and return this mash to the remaining beans.
13. Place the cooking pot on the stove and heat olive oil in it.
14. Add the carrots and onion. Sauté for 7 minutes, then add the garlic.
15. Cook for 1 minute, then add the rosemary, pepper, bean mixture, and stock.
16. Allow the mixture to cool, then boil it and reduce the heat to a simmer.

17. Let it simmer for 5 more minutes.
18. Serve the soup with the croutons on top.
19. Garnish with a rosemary sprig and enjoy.

Serving Suggestion: Serve the soup with a bowl of potato salad.

Variation Tip: Add a small drop of hot sauce for some kick.

Nutritional Information per Serving:
Calories 301 | Fat 6g |Sodium 62mg | Carbs 24g | Fiber 0.2g | Sugar 1g | Protein 16g

Barley Tomato Risotto

Prep Time: 10 minutes
Cook Time: 1 hour and 20 minutes
Serves: 4
Ingredients:
- 10 large plum tomatoes, peeled and chopped
- 2 tablespoons olive oil
- ½ teaspoon black pepper
- 4 cups vegetable stock
- 3 cups water
- 2 cups pearl barley
- 2 shallots, chopped
- ¼ cup dry white wine
- 3 tablespoons fresh basil, chopped
- 3 tablespoons fresh parsley, chopped
- 1½ tablespoons fresh thyme, chopped
- ½ cup parmesan cheese, grated

Preparation:
1. Preheat the oven to 450°F.
2. Spread the tomatoes on a baking sheet and toss them with the salt, pepper, and oil.
3. Roast them in the oven for 30 minutes and keep 16 wedges for garnishing.
4. Mix the stock with the water and boil on high heat.
5. Reduce the heat to a simmer.
6. Add 1 tablespoon of oil to a saucepan and heat it.
7. Stir in the shallots and sauté for 3 minutes, then add the white wine.
8. Cook for 3 minutes, then add the barley.
9. Stir cook for 1 minute and add ½ cup stock mixture.
10. Cook until the liquid is completely absorbed.
11. Continue adding the stock mixture while cooking the barley for 50 minutes in total.
12. Turn off the stove and stir in the tomatoes, basil, thyme, cheese, parsley, basil, and tomatoes.
13. Serve.

Serving Suggestion: Serve the risotto with a bowl of Greek salad.
Variation Tip: Add chopped herbs on top.
Nutritional Information per Serving:
Calories 240 | Fat 7.4g |Sodium 120mg | Carbs 45g |
Fiber 0.2g | Sugar 1g | Protein 6.2g

Crispy Coconut Shrimp

Prep Time: 10 minutes
Cook Time: 15 minutes
Serves: 4
Ingredients:
• ¼ cup unsweetened coconut
• ¼ cup Panko breadcrumbs
• ½ teaspoon Kosher salt
• ½ cup coconut milk
• 12 large shrimp, peeled and deveined
Preparation:
1. Switch on the oven and set it to 375° F to preheat.
2. Grease a baking pan with cooking spray and set it aside. Grind Panko with salt and coconut in a food processor.
3. Add this mixture to a bowl and pour coconut milk into another bowl.
4. First, dip each shrimp in coconut milk, then coat it with Panko mixture.
5. Place the coated shrimp in the baking pan. Cover them with a light layer of cooking spray.
6. Bake for 15 minutes.
7. Serve warm.
Serving Suggestion: Serve with low-sodium tomato sauce.
Variation Tip: Substitute Panko breadcrumbs with whole wheat breadcrumbs.
Nutritional Information per Serving:
Calories 249 | Fat 11.9 g | Sodium 77 mg | Carbs 1.8 g | Fiber 1.2 g | Sugar 0.3 g | Protein 35 g

Tomato Basil Halibut

Prep Time: 15 minutes
Cook Time: 12 minutes
Serves: 4
Ingredients:
• 2 tomatoes, diced
• 2 tablespoons fresh basil, chopped
• 1 teaspoon fresh oregano, chopped
• 1 tablespoon garlic, minced
• 2 teaspoons olive oil
• 4 halibut fillets
Preparation:
1. Preheat the oven to 350°F.
2. Layer a 9-inch x 13-inch baking pan with cooking spray.
3. Toss the tomato with basil, olive oil, garlic, and oregano in a bowl.
4. Place the halibut fillets in the baking pan and pour the tomato mixture on top.
5. Bake for 12 minutes until the fish is done.
6. Serve.
Serving Suggestion: Serve the fish with a bowl of roasted asparagus salad.
Variation Tip: Add chopped herbs on top.
Nutritional Information per Serving:
Calories 205 | Fat 20g |Sodium 41mg | Carbs 6.1g | Fiber 0.9g | Sugar 0.9g | Protein 22g

Lime Braised Cauliflower

Prep Time: 10 minutes
Cook Time: 20 minutes
Serves: 4
Ingredients:
• 1 medium head cauliflower, cored and chopped into 1½-inch florets
• ⅓ cup chicken broth
• 2 tablespoons minced fresh parsley
• Juice from 1 large lime
• 3 tablespoons olive oil
• ⅛ teaspoon red pepper, sliced
• 3 garlic cloves, minced
• Salt and pepper, to taste
Preparation:
1. Mix 1 teaspoon oil, garlic and pepper in a small bowl.
2. Heat remaining three tablespoons oil in a large skillet over medium-high heat until glistening and shimmering.
3. Whisk in cauliflower and ¼ teaspoon salt and cook, stirring from time to time, until florets become golden brown, 7 to 9 minutes.
4. Move cauliflower to sides of skillet. Pour garlic mixture to center and continue to cook, crushing mixture into skillet, until garlic begins to sizzle about 30 seconds.

5. Combine garlic mixture into cauliflower and mix well with a wire whisk.

6. Pour in broth and lime juice and bring to simmer. Reduce heat to medium-low, cover and cook until cauliflower is crisp-tender, 4 to 6 minutes.

7. Remove from the heat, and sprinkle with salt and pepper to season.

8. Serve.

Serving Suggestion: Stir in parsley.

Variation Tip: For vibrancy, use a teaspoon of smoked paprika.

Nutritional Information per Serving:
Calories 72 | Fat 4.9g | Sodium 166mg | Carbs 4.2g | Fiber 1.4g | Sugar 1.52g | Protein 3.19g

Glazed Chicken Skewers

Prep Time: 10 minutes
Cook Time: 8 minutes
Serves: 4
Ingredients:
- 12 skewers
- 4 (4 ounces, 113g) chicken breasts, cut into 1-inch cubes
- 3 large red bell peppers, cut into 1-inch pieces
- 2 large white onions, cut into 1-inch pieces
- 6 apricots, pitted and cut into 1-inch pieces

Marinade:
- 1 heaping tablespoon reduced-sugar apricot marmalade
- ½ teaspoon sesame oil
- ¼ cup extra virgin olive oil
- 1 ½ teaspoon finely chopped fresh ginger
- 1 tablespoon Dijon mustard or brown mustard
- 4 tablespoons apple cider vinegar
- 1 large clove garlic, chopped

Preparation:
1. Mix all marinade ingredients in a large bowl.
2. Place the cubed chicken in a large zip-top bag, pour in the marinade, squeeze the air out of the bag, and seal tightly.
3. Work the mixture into the chicken by hand by moving the bag and contents around. Let the chicken marinate in the refrigerator for at least two hours if you can.
4. Soak 12 large wooden skewers in water, and then chop the peppers, onions and apricots into similar-sized pieces.
5. Skewer the pieces of chicken, pepper, onion, and apricot, alternating ingredients.
6. Grill the skewers on a hot grill or grill pan, about 4 to 5 minutes per side, or until the chicken is no longer pink in the center.

Serving Suggestion: Serve alongside a salad of your choice.

Variation Tip: Substitute the fresh ginger with ¾ teaspoon ground ginger.

Nutritional Information per Serving:
Calories 314 | Fat 16 g | Sodium 357 mg | Carbs 21 g | Fiber 4 g | Sugar 10 g | Protein 25 g

Tomato Peach Soup

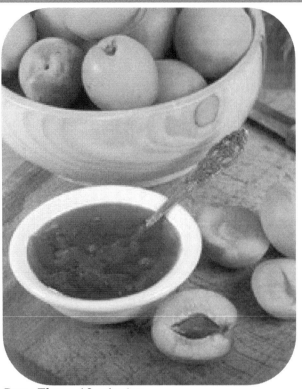

Prep Time: 10 minutes
Cook Time: 12 minutes
Serves: 4
Ingredients:
- ½ tablespoon olive oil
- 1 large ripe peach, halved, pitted, peeled and diced
- 1 cup carrots, shredded
- 2 garlic cloves, minced
- 1 can no-salt diced tomatoes in juice
- ½ teaspoon chili pepper, freshly ground
- 1 cup chicken broth, low-sodium
- 1 cup water
- 1 cup yogurt

Preparation:
1. Heat the olive oil in a large pot over medium heat.
2. Add the shredded carrots and cook, often stirring, about 5 minutes, or until carrots are tender. Sprinkle with garlic, and cook for 1 minute.
3. Remove the carrot mixture to a food processor.
4. Add the tomatoes and their juice, broth, chili pepper and water, and purée until smooth.
5. Return the purée to the pot, reduce heat to medium-low, cook the soup mixture for 5 minutes, or cook until cooked through.
6. Smear with the yogurt.
7. Enjoy.

Serving Suggestion: Garnish each serving with a quarter of the peach slices.

Variation Tip: Low-fat buttermilk is used in place of heavy cream in this recipe, creating a rich soup.

Nutritional Information per Serving:
Calories 155 | Fat 9g | Sodium 116mg | Carbs 17g | Fiber 5g | Sugar 4g | Protein 5g

Baked Lamb Meatballs

Prep Time: 10 minutes
Cook Time: 20 minutes
Serves: 4
Ingredients:
• 1 pound ground lamb
• Olive oil cooking spray
• 1 large egg, beaten
• 1 garlic clove, chopped
• ¼ cup fresh mint, chopped
• ¼ cup shallot, chopped
• ¼ teaspoon ground cinnamon
• ½ teaspoon Kosher salt
• ¼ teaspoon red pepper flakes
• 1 teaspoon ground coriander
• 1 teaspoon ground cumin
Preparation:
1. Preheat the oven to 400° F. Grease a 12-cup muffin tin with olive oil cooking spray.
2. Mix the lamb, mint, egg, garlic, shallot, salt, coriander, cinnamon, cumin and red pepper flakes; stir well.
3. Shape the batter into 12 balls and put one in each cup of the prepared muffin tin.
4. Air-fry for 20 minutes, or until the meatballs are golden brown.
5. Remove from the oven and serve on plates.
Serving Suggestion: You can serve these lamb meatballs with whole-wheat pita and Tzatziki.
Variation Tip: Ground beef or poultry can be used in place of the lamb if preferred.
Nutritional Information per Serving:
Calories 350 | Fat 28g | Sodium 227mg | Carbs 2g | Fiber 1g | Sugar 0g | Protein 21g

Chicken Stew

Prep Time: 10 minutes
Cook Time: 30 minutes
Serves: 5
Ingredients:

• 1-pound boneless, skinless chicken breasts, cut into 1-inch cubes (2.5 cm)
• 1 ½ cups peeled, cubed potatoes
• ½ cup sliced celery
• ½ cup chopped onions
• ½ cup thinly sliced carrots
• ¼ teaspoon pepper
• ½ teaspoon paprika
• ¼ teaspoon dried thyme
• ¼ teaspoon rubbed sage
• 3 ounces unsalted tomato paste
• 1 ½ tablespoons cornstarch mixed with two tablespoons water
• 1 can (14.5 ounces) low-sodium chicken broth
• Shredded Parmesan cheese, to serve (optional)
Preparation:
1. Place chicken, vegetables, spices, herbs, tomato paste and broth in a soup pot. Stir until well combined.
2. Cook covered over medium flame until chicken and vegetables are tender.
3. Add cornstarch mixture and constantly stir until thick.
4. Ladle into bowls and serve.
Serving Suggestion: Garnish with parmesan if using.
Variation Tip: Substitute chicken broth with low sodium beef broth.
Nutritional Information per Serving:
Calories 180 | Fat 2g | Sodium 280mg | Carbs 18g | Fiber 4g | Sugar 6g | Protein 21g

Roasted Pork Loin and Potatoes

Prep Time: 10 minutes
Cook Time: 1 hour
Serves: 4
Ingredients:
• 1 (1-pound/454-gram) pork loin, trimmed
• 8 garlic cloves
• ¼ cup olive oil, divided
• Black pepper, to taste
• 1 cup cubed raw sweet potato
• 1 cup small gold potatoes, quartered
• 8 fresh thyme sprigs, chopped
Preparation:
1. Preheat the oven to 350° F.
2. Rub the pork with garlic and 2 tablespoons of olive oil.
3. Season with black pepper. Coat a 9-by-13-inch baking dish with nonstick cooking spray.
4. Place the pork in the prepared baking dish.
5. Bake for an hour, or until an instant-read thermometer inserted in the center registers 145° F.
6. Twenty minutes into the cooking time, place the cubed and sliced sweet potatoes and gold potatoes on a rimmed baking dish, drizzle with the remaining olive oil, sprinkle with the thyme, and place in the oven.

7. The potatoes should be finished roasting about the same time as the pork and should be tender and slightly browned.

8. Once the pork is finished cooking, remove it from the oven and let the meat stand for 15 minutes before carving.

9. Cut into eight slices.

Serving Suggestion: Serve with roasted potatoes and a green salad.

Variation Tip: Dried thyme can be used in place of fresh thyme.

Nutritional Information per Serving:
Calories 426 | Fat 22 g | Sodium 56 mg | Carbs 21 g | Fiber 4 g | Sugar 3 g | Protein 27 g

Grilled Flank Steak with Peach Compote

Prep Time: 10 minutes
Cook Time: 25 minutes
Serves: 6
Ingredients:
Peach Compote:
• 2 peaches, cored and diced
• 1 tablespoon honey
• ½ tablespoon apple cider vinegar
• ¼ teaspoon ground cinnamon
• ¼ teaspoon ground ginger
• ¼ teaspoon ground nutmeg
• ¼ teaspoon Kosher or Sea salt
Grilled Flank Steak:
• 1½ pounds flank steak
• 2 tablespoons canola oil
• ½ teaspoon Kosher or Sea salt
• ¼ teaspoon ground black pepper
Preparation:
Make the Peach Compote:
1. Place the peaches, honey, apple cider vinegar, cinnamon, ginger, nutmeg and salt in a saucepan and bring to a simmer.
2. Stirring frequently, cook for 7 to 10 minutes, until the peaches are tender and the mixture has thickened. Remove from the heat and reserve.
Make the Grilled Flank Steak:
3. Heat a grill or grill pan over medium-high heat. Coat the steak with canola oil, salt and black pepper.
4. Grill for 6 minutes per side until the internal temperature reaches 155º F.
5. Let rest for 10 minutes on a cutting board, then thinly slice across the grain.
6. Divide the steak and serve.
Serving Suggestion: Serve with the peach compote.
Variation Tip: Replace honey with a no-calorie sweetener of your choice.
Nutritional Information per Serving:

Calories 236 | Fat 12 g | Sodium 356 mg | Carbs 7 g | Fiber 1 g | Sugar 5 g | Protein 24 g

Spicy Bean Chili

Prep Time: 10 minutes
Cook Time: 20 minutes
Serves: 2
Ingredients:
• 1 teaspoon of grapeseed oil
• ½ medium size red onion
• ½ Jalapeno pepper
• 1 garlic clove
• 15 ounces of low sodium red kidney beans
• ¾ cups of vegetable broth (low sodium)
• 3 fresh medium tomatoes (chopped)
• ¾ teaspoons chili powder
• ¼ teaspoon of sea salt
• ⅛ teaspoon of ground cinnamon
Preparation:
1. Warm oil in a saucepan with medium-high heat.
2. Add the onion and Jalapeño, after which you sauté for 5 minutes till the onion is caramelized.
3. Put the garlic and sauté until fragrant for about 30 seconds.
4. Add the rest of the ingredients and stir. Allow them to a boil 1 minute warmly.
5. Cover with the lid and simmer in medium heat for 10 minutes until well combined.
6. Enjoy.
Serving Suggestion: Garnish with fresh coriander or organic low-fat sour cream.
Variation Tip: Feel free to use olive oil in place of grapeseed oil.
Nutritional Information per Serving:
Calories 270 | Fat 2g | Sodium 790mg | Carbs 45g | Fiber 17g | Sugar 5g | Protein 17g

Cheesy Pasta Bake

Prep Time: 10 minutes
Cook Time: 35 minutes
Serves: 8
Ingredients:

- 1 ¼ cups whole-grain pasta
- 1 head Romanesco cauliflower, cut into florets
- 2 tablespoons olive oil
- 1 tablespoon corn flour
- 2 cups low fat milk
- 1 teaspoon hot English mustard
- Olive oil cooking spray
- 1 cup grated homemade Gouda cheese
- 1 cup grated Emmental cheese
- Black pepper to taste
- ¼ cup coarsely ground almonds
- ½ teaspoon ground paprika

Preparation:
1. Bring a pot of water to a boil and cook the pasta for about 7 minutes.
2. At the same time, bring a smaller pot of water to a boil, and cook the cauliflower florets for about 5 minutes.
3. Drain both the pasta and cauliflower and set aside.
4. Preheat the oven to 350º F. Next, make the sauce. Heat the oil in a medium pot, then whisk in the corn flour, being sure to remove any lumps that form.
5. Gradually add in the milk, whisking all the time to prevent lumps from forming. Lastly, mix in the mustard and let the sauce come to a boil.
6. Then add the grated Gouda and Emmental, whisk until they melt, and remove from the heat. Add the pasta and cauliflower into the saucepot and stir well.
7. Add black pepper to taste. Pour the pasta mixture into an oiled casserole dish, and top with the ground almonds.
8. Sprinkle over some paprika and bake in the oven for about 20 minutes until the sauce starts to bubble on the sides.
9. Rest the dish for 5 minutes, then serve hot.

Serving Suggestion: Garnish with parsley.

Variation Tip: You can swap out the ground almonds for Panko breadcrumbs and the cheeses for any cheese you like. This dish is also great, using Macaroni instead of pasta screws.

Nutritional Information per Serving:
Calories 234 | Fat 10g | Sodium 88mg | Carbs 23g | Fiber 2g | Sugar 5g | Protein 13g

Sweet and Sour Cabbage with Pork Chops

Prep Time: 10 minutes
Cook Time: 1 hour 10 minutes
Serves: 4
Ingredients:
Sweet and Sour Cabbage:
- 1 tablespoon olive oil
- 1 medium red onion, sliced
- 2 rashers low sodium back bacon, cut into cubes
- ½ medium-sized white cabbage, sliced

- ¼ cup white grape vinegar
- 3 tablespoon golden syrup
- ¼ cup water
- 2 crisp green apples, peeled and diced
- Black pepper to taste

Pork Chops:
- Olive oil cooking spray
- 4, 4 ounces pork chops, fat removed
- Black pepper to taste

Preparation:
1. Heat the oil in a pan, add the onion and fry for 1 minute. Then add the bacon pieces and cook until crispy and browned.
2. Add ⅓ of the cabbage, and sprinkle over ⅓ of the vinegar.
3. Repeat this process until the cabbage and vinegar are all incorporated. Then add the syrup, water, apples, and black pepper and reduce the heat. Leave to simmer on low for about 1 hour.
4. Ten minutes before the cabbage is ready, heat and oil a nonstick pan.
5. Place the pork chops in the pan and fry until golden brown on each side, about 3 minutes aside.
6. While cooking, add black pepper to taste. Set aside covered to keep warm.
7. Transfer the cabbage mixture to the hot chops pan and stir well on high for 3 minutes.
8. Enjoy.

Serving Suggestion: To serve, use a slotted spoon. To avoid getting juices on the plate, spoon the cabbage mixture neatly onto the center of the plate and place the hot chops on top.

Variation Tip: Replace water with low sodium vegetable broth.

Nutritional Information per Serving:
Calories 356 | Fat 10g | Sodium 377mg | Carbs 39g | Fiber 6g | Sugar 8g | Protein 29g

Cajun Baked Trout

Prep Time: 10 minutes
Cook Time: 15 minutes
Serves: 4
Ingredients:
- ¼ teaspoon chili powder
- 1 teaspoon Treacle sugar
- 1 teaspoon brown onion powder
- 1 teaspoon paprika powder
- 2 teaspoon dried parsley
- 1 teaspoon dried oregano
- 1 teaspoon garlic powder
- 1 teaspoon ground cumin
- Black pepper to taste
- 17 ounces broccoli florets
- 4, 6 ounces Rainbow trout fillets
- 1 teaspoon olive oil
- 1 lemon, cut into four pieces

Preparation:

1. Make the crust for the fish by mixing all the dried spices and herbs in a bowl.
2. Lightly oil the fish fillets and then pat the spice crust onto them evenly. Place them on a well-oiled baking tray.
3. Preheat the oven to 425º F and lightly oil a baking tray.
4. Dress the broccoli with a little olive oil and pepper and place on the second oiled baking tray.
5. Bake both trays in the oven simultaneously, for about 12-15 minutes, or until the fish and broccoli are superbly cooked.
6. The trout should pull apart effortlessly and have a crisp, dark crust.

Serving Suggestion: Serve with lemon quarters for squeezing.

Variation Tip: You can easily replace the trout in this recipe with salmon.

Nutritional Information per Serving:
Calories 280 | Fat 11g | Sodium 227mg | Carbs 10g | Fiber 4g | Sugar 7g | Protein 38g

Veggie Pita Rolls

Prep Time: 15 minutes
Serves: 1
Ingredients:
- ½ bell pepper, seeded and chopped
- ½ tomato, seeded and chopped
- ½ garlic clove, minced finely
- ¼ tablespoon fresh lime juice
- 1 whole-wheat pita bread, warmed
- ½ cup romaine lettuce, shredded
- ½ red onion, chopped
- ¼ cup cucumber, chopped
- ½ tablespoon olive oil
- Fresh ground black pepper to flavor

Preparation:
1. Take a bowl and include all the above ingredients except for pita bread and gently toss to coat well.
2. Place pita bread onto the serving plate.
3. Top it with salad and roll the pita bread.
4. Serve and enjoy!

Serving Suggestions: Serve it with Tzatziki sauce or your favorite kind of sauce.

Variation Tip: You can also enjoy it with olives.

Nutritional Information per Serving:
Calories: 340 | Fat: 11.8g | Sat Fat: 1.7g | Carbohydrates: 53.5g | Fiber: 9.3g | Sugar: 7.6g | Protein: 10.6g

Arugula Quinoa Risotto

Prep Time: 15 minutes
Cook Time: 20 minutes
Serves: 6
Ingredients:
- 1 tablespoon olive oil
- ½ cup yellow onion, chopped
- 1 garlic clove, minced
- 1 cup quinoa, rinsed
- 2¼ cups low-sodium vegetable stock
- 2 cups arugula, chopped and stemmed
- 1 small carrot, peeled and shredded
- ½ cup shiitake mushrooms, sliced
- ¼ cup parmesan cheese, grated
- ¼ teaspoon salt
- ¼ teaspoon ground black pepper

Preparation:
1. Add the oil to a saucepan, then heat it.
2. Stir in the onion and sauté for 4 minutes until soft.
3. Add the quinoa and garlic. Cook for 1 minute.
4. Stir in the stock and bring it to a boil, then reduce the heat to a simmer.
5. Cook for 12 minutes until the quinoa is al dente.
6. Add the carrot, mushrooms, and arugula.
7. Cook for another two minutes.
8. Add salt, pepper, and cheese.
9. Serve warm.

Serving Suggestion: Serve the risotto with a bowl of roasted cauliflower salad.

Variation Tip: Season the risotto with some dried herbs.

Nutritional Information per Serving:
Calories 288 | Fat 5.1g | Sodium 64mg | Carbs 28g | Fiber 3.9g | Sugar 1.4g | Protein 6g

Tofu & Oats Burgers

Prep Time: 8 minutes
Cook Time: 16 minutes
Serves: 2
Ingredients:
- 6 tablespoons rolled oats
- 2 garlic cloves, minced
- ½ medium onion, finely chopped

- 1 cup frozen spinach, thawed
- 2 tablespoons flaxseeds
- ½ pound firm drained, pressed and crumbled
- ½ teaspoon red pepper flakes, crushed
- 1 tablespoon olive oil
- Fresh ground black pepper to taste
- ½ teaspoon ground cumin
- 3 cups fresh salad greens

Preparation:
1. Take a bowl and include all the above ingredients except for olive-oil and salad greens and mix them all together until well combined.
2. Set aside the bowl for about ten minutes.
3. Make patties from the prepared mixture.
4. Now, take a non-stick frying pan and heat the oil over medium heat.
5. Cook the patties for about six to eight minutes each side.
6. Serve and enjoy!

Serving Suggestions: Serve the patties alongside salad greens and ketchup.
Variation Tip: You can use your favorite veggies.
Nutritional Information per Serving:

Calories: 309 | Fat: 15.2g | Sat Fat: 2.5g | Carbohydrates: 29.4g | Fiber: 10.1g | Sugar: 2.3g | Protein: 18.2g

Cauliflower & Peas Curry

Prep Time: 20 minutes
Cook Time: 15 minutes
Serves: 6
Ingredients:
- ½ cup water
- 4 medium tomatoes, chopped
- 4 cup cauliflower, chopped
- 4 tablespoons olive oil
- 6 garlic cloves, minced
- 2 teaspoons Cayenne pepper
- 2 teaspoons ground cumin
- 2 teaspoons ground coriander
- 1 tablespoon fresh ginger, minced
- ½ teaspoon ground turmeric
- 2 cup fresh green peas, shelled
- Fresh ground black pepper to taste
- Pinch of salt
- 1 cup warm water

Preparation:
1. Take a food processor, add tomatoes and half cup of water and pulse until you have a smooth puree.
2. Set aside the formed mixture.
3. In a large saucepan, heat the oil over medium heat and fry the garlic, green chilies and spices for about a minute.
4. Add the cauliflower, peas and tomato puree to the pan and cook for about three to four minutes.
5. Now, pour warm water and bring it to a boil.

6. Reduce the heat to medium-low and let it cook for about eight to ten minutes while covered.
Serving Suggestions: Serve it with some rice.
Variation Tip: You can also add other veggies like cubed potato, root veggies etc.
Nutritional Information per Serving:
Calories: 163 | Fat: 10.1g | Sat Fat: 1.5g | Carbohydrates: 16.1g | Fiber: 5.6g | Sugar: 6.7g | Protein: 5.1g

Veggie Ratatouille

Prep Time: 15 minutes
Cook Time: 45 minutes
Serves: 2
Ingredients:
- 1½ tablespoons olive oil, divided
- 6 tablespoons garlic, minced
- ½ zucchini, sliced into thin circles
- ½ eggplant, thinly sliced into circles
- ½ tablespoon fresh thyme leaves, minced
- ½ tablespoon fresh lemon juice
- 1 red bell pepper, seeded and thinly-sliced into circles
- ¾ cup water
- ½ yellow squash, thinly sliced into circles
- ¼ onion, chopped
- ⅜ cup salt-free tomato paste
- Pinch of salt
- Fresh ground black pepper to taste

Preparation:
1. Preheat the oven to 375° F.
2. Take a bowl, add the tomato paste, oil, onion, garlic, salt and black pepper and blend them well all together.
3. In the base of a baking dish, spread the tomato paste mixture evenly.
4. Arrange alternating vegetable slices, starting at the outer edge of the baking dish and working concentrically towards the center.
5. Drizzle the vegetables with the remaining oil and sprinkle with salt and black pepper.

6. Arrange a piece of parchment paper over the vegetables.
7. Bake them about 45 minutes.
8. Serve them hot.
9. Enjoy!
Serving Suggestions: Serve it with cooked eggs.
Variation Tip: Peel the eggplants and salt them to remove their water.
Nutritional Information per Serving:
Calories: 239 | Fat: 1.6g | Sat Fat: 1.6g |
Carbohydrates: 34.1g | Fiber: 9.1g | Sugar: 14.9g |
Protein: 6.6g

Kidney Beans Curry

Prep Time: 10 minutes
Cook Time: 25 minutes
Serves: 2
Ingredients:
- 1 cup water
- 1 large plum tomato, chopped finely
- ⅛ teaspoon Cayenne pepper
- ½ teaspoon ground cumin
- ½ cup low-sodium tomato sauce
- ½ garlic cloves, minced
- ⅛ cup olive oil
- 1½ cup cooked red kidney beans
- ¼ cup fresh parsley, chopped
- ¼ teaspoon ground turmeric
- ½ teaspoon ground coriander
- 1 tablespoon fresh ginger, minced
- ½ medium onion, chopped finely
- Fresh ground black pepper to taste
Preparation:
1. Grab a large frying pan and heat oil over medium heat and fry onion, garlic and ginger for about four to five minutes.
2. Stir in tomato sauce and spices and cook for about five minutes.
3. Stir in tomatoes, kidney beans and water and bring it to a boil over high heat.
4. Lessen the heat to medium and gently cook for about ten to 15 minutes or until we have the desired thickness.
5. Serve hot and enjoy!
Serving Suggestions: Garnish parsley before serving.
Variation Tip: You can also add your favorite vegetables such as mushrooms, broccoli or potatoes.
Nutritional Information per Serving:
Calories: 628 | Fat: 14.6g | Sat Fat: 2.1g |
Carbohydrates: 96.1g | Fiber: 23.8g | Sugar: 8.4g |
Protein: 33.4g

Chicken Kabobs

Prep Time: 10 minutes
Cook Time: 8 minutes
Serves: 2
Ingredients:
- 1 tablespoon olive oil
- ⅛ teaspoon Cayenne pepper
- ½ garlic clove, pepper
- 6 tablespoons fat-free plain Greek yogurt
- 1 tablespoon ground cumin
- 1 tablespoon fresh lemon juice
- 2 boneless chicken-breasts, cut into 1-inch chunks
- Pinch of salt
- Fresh ground black pepper according to your flavor
Preparation:
1. Take a bowl and add all the ingredients except for chicken chunks and mix them until well combined.
2. Add the chicken chunks and coat with the yogurt mixture generously.
3. Refrigerate overnight.
4. Preheat the grill to medium-high heat and grease the grill grate finely.
5. Thread the chicken chunks onto pre-soaked wooden skewers.
6. Arrange chicken kabobs onto the grill and cook for about three to four minutes per side.
7. Serve hot and enjoy!
Serving Suggestions: Serve it with your favorite sauce or ketchup.
Variation Tip: Try to cut all the chicken pieces of same size.
Nutritional Information per Serving:
Calories: 221 | Fat: 9.3g | Sat Fat: 1.1g |
Carbohydrates: 3.7g | Fiber: 0.4g | Sugar: 1.9g |
Protein: 31.2g

Mango Tortillas

Prep Time: 15 minutes
Serves: 2
Ingredients:
- 2 whole-wheat tortillas, warmed
- ½ cup purple cabbage, shredded
- ½ tablespoon Dijon mustard
- 1 tablespoon fresh lime juice
- ½ cup mango, peeled, pitted and cubed
- ⅛ cup fresh cilantro, chopped
- 1 tablespoon olive oil
- Fresh ground black pepper to taste

Preparation:
1. Take a large bowl, add mustard, lime juice, oil and black pepper and beat until well combined.
2. Add mango, cabbage and cilantro and toss them all to coat well.
3. Arrange the tortillas onto a smooth surface.
4. Place mixture over each tortilla, leaving about one inch border all around.
5. Carefully fold the edges of each tortilla over the filling to roll up.
6. Cut each roll in half cross-wise.
7. Serve and enjoy!

Serving Suggestions: Serve with black beans on the side.
Variation Tip: You can also use a drained tin of sliced mangoes.
Nutritional Information per Serving:
Calories: 229 | Fat: 10.7g | Sat Fat: 2.2g | Carbohydrates: 20g| Fiber: 2.9g | Sugar: 6.8g | Protein: 15.1g

Red Beans and Rice

Prep Time: 10 minutes
Cook Time: 45 minutes
Serves: 2
Ingredients:
- ½ cup dry brown rice
- 1 cup water, plus ¼ cup
- 1 (15 ounces) can of red beans, drained and rinsed
- 1 tablespoon ground cumin
- Juice of 1 lime
- 4 handfuls of fresh spinach
- Optional toppings: avocado, chopped tomatoes, Greek yogurt, onions

Preparation:
1. Combine rice and water in a pot and bring to a boil. Cover and reduce heat to a low simmer.
2. Cook for 30 to 40 minutes or according to package directions.
3. Meanwhile, add the beans, ¼ cup of water, cumin and lime juice to a medium skillet. Bring to a boil. Reduce to a simmer and let cook until most of the liquid is absorbed 5 to 7 minutes.
4. Once the liquid is mostly gone, remove it from the heat and add spinach.
5. Cover and let spinach wilt slightly, 2 to 3 minutes. Mix in with the beans.

Serving Suggestion: Serve beans with rice. Add toppings if using.
Variation Tip: Keep your freezer stocked with an assortment of frozen vegetables, including spinach, broccoli, cauliflower, summer squash and peppers. Add your favorites to boost the fiber and vitamins and minerals in this recipe.
Nutritional Information per Serving:
Calories 232 | Fat 2g | Sodium 210mg | Carbs 41g | Fiber 12g | Sugar 1g | Protein 13g

Curried Cod

Prep Time: 10 minutes
Cook Time: 25 minutes
Serves: 2
Ingredients:
- ½ tablespoon oil
- 1 tablespoon curry powder
- 2 cloves garlic, crushed
- ½ can (from 14.1 ounces can) chickpeas
- Zest of ½ lemon, grated
- ½ onion, chopped
- 1 inch (2.5 cm) ginger, peeled, finely grated
- 1 can (14.1 ounces) chopped tomatoes
- 2 Cod fillets (about 5 ounces)
- Chopped cilantro to garnish
- Lemon wedges to serve
- Salt to taste

Preparation:
1. Place a pan (that has a fitting lid) over medium flame. Pour oil into the pan and let it heat.
2. Once the oil is heated, stir in onions and cook until translucent.
3. Add ginger, garlic and curry powder and cook for a couple of minutes until you get a nice aroma.
4. Add tomatoes and mix well. Cook for a couple of minutes, stirring often.

5. Stir in chickpeas and salt. Cook until slightly thick. Place Cod in the pan and cover the pan with a fitting lid.

6. Once the fish is cooked, turn off the heat.

7. Serve and enjoy.

Serving Suggestion: Garnish with lemon zest, lemon wedges, and cilantro and serve.

Variation Tip: Use two large tomatoes in place of the canned tomatoes.

Nutritional Information per Serving:

Calories 296 | Fat 6g | Sodium 757mg | Carbs 22g | Fiber10.5g | Sugar 1.4g| Protein 34g

Couscous with Veggies

Prep Time: 8 minutes

Cook Time: 15 minutes

Serves: 2

Ingredients:
- 1 garlic clove, minced
- ½ cup pearl couscous
- ½ shallot, chopped
- ½ teaspoon Balsamic vinegar
- 1 tablespoon olive oil, divided
- ½ tablespoon fresh lemon juice
- 1 cup cauliflower florets
- 3/2 tablespoon dates, pitted and chopped
- 1 tablespoon fresh parsley, chopped
- ⅝ cup low-sodium vegetable broth
- Fresh ground black pepper to taste

Preparation:

1. For couscous: Take a large pan and heat one tablespoon of oil over medium-heat and fry the garlic for about one minute.

2. Add the broth and couscous to the pan and continue stirring.

3. Reduce the heat to medium and gently cook for about eight to ten minutes.

4. Stir in the lemon juice and remove the pan from the heat.

5. Take a pan and heat the remaining oil over medium heat and fry the shallot for about two minutes.

6. Stir in the cauliflower and cook for about five to six minutes.

7. Stir in the dates and cook for about another two minutes.

8. Add vinegar and black pepper and remove the pan from the heat.

9. Transfer the cauliflower mixture into the pan with couscous and stir to combine everything very well.

Serving Suggestions: Serve warm with the garnishing of parsley.

Variation Tip: Try to cook the couscous mixture until steam begin to emerge.

Nutritional Information per Serving:

Calories: 266 | Fat: 7.5g | Sat Fat: 1g | Carbohydrates: 43g | Fiber: 2g | Sugar: 6.6g | Protein: 7.4g

Citrus Beef Stir Fry

Prep Time: 10 minutes

Cook Time: 10 minutes

Serves: 2

Ingredients:
- ½ pound boneless beef sirloin steak, cut into thin strips
- 2 teaspoons olive oil, divided
- ¼ cup orange juice
- 1 tablespoon reduced-sodium soy sauce
- 1 tablespoon cornstarch
- ¼ cup cold water
- 3 cups frozen stir-fry vegetable blend
- 1 garlic clove, minced

Preparation:

1. Mix the cornstarch, water, orange juice and soy sauce until smooth in a small bowl. Set the mixture aside.

2. In a large wok or skillet, heat one teaspoon of olive oil over medium-high heat.

3. Stir-fry the beef for 3 to 4 minutes, until no longer pink.

4. Remove to a plate or bowl and cover to keep warm.

5. Add the remaining olive oil to the wok and allow to heat. Stir-fry the vegetable blend and garlic for 3 minutes.

6. Stir the cornstarch mixture, then add it to the cooking vegetables and bring to a boil. Stir for 2 minutes, until thickened.

7. Add the beef and stir until heated through.

Serving Suggestion: Top with sesame seeds.

Variation Tip: You can reduce the beef by half and add in 1 cup of frozen protein-rich edamame. This would also help you practice taking the focus off meat and making the meal more plant-based.

Nutritional Information per Serving:

Calories 268 | Fat 10g | Sodium 376mg | Carbs 8g | Fiber 3g | Sugar 8g | Protein 26g

Veggies Stuffed Bell Peppers

Prep Time: 10 minutes
Cook Time: 25 minutes
Serves: 2
Ingredients:
- ¼ pound fresh shiitake mushrooms
- 1 tablespoon olive oil
- 1 garlic cloves, peeled
- 2 bell peppers, halved and seeded
- ½ cup celery stalk
- ¼ cup unsalted walnuts
- Pinch of salt
- Fresh ground black pepper to taste

Preparation:
1. Preheat oven to 400° F.
2. Evenly grease the baking sheet.
3. Remove stem and seeds from bell peppers.
4. In a food processor, add mushrooms, celery, garlic, walnuts, oil, salt, pepper and pulse until everything is chopped finely.
5. Stuff the prepared mushroom mixture into the bell peppers.
6. Arrange the bell peppers onto the baking sheet.
7. Bake them about 20-25 minutes or until they are slightly brown.
8. Serve warm.

Serving Suggestions: Top the peppers with parsley.
Variation Tip: You can also use green peppers instead.
Nutritional Information per Serving:
Calories: 138 | Fat: 7.8g | Sat Fat: 1.1g | Carbohydrates: 18.2g | Fiber: 3.3g | Sugar: 8.4g | Protein: 2.4g

Tomato & Feta Salad

Prep Time: 15 minutes
Serves: 2
Ingredients:
- 1 large fresh tomato, sliced
- ½ tablespoon olive oil

- 1 scallions, chopped
- 1½ tablespoon Feta cheese, crumbled
- 3 cups fresh baby greens
- ½ red onion, sliced
- 1 tablespoon unsalted almonds, chopped
- 1 tablespoon fresh lemon-juice

Preparation:
1. Take a bowl and add all the given ingredients except for almonds and cheese and toss to coat well.
2. Cover and refrigerate to let it sit and marinate for about six to eight hours.
3. Remove from the refrigerator and stir in the almonds.
4. Serve with the topping of Feta cheese.

Serving Suggestions: Serve it with the sprinkle of herbs.
Variation Tip: You can also add fresh chopped basil.
Nutritional Information per Serving:
Calories: 150 | Fat: 6.8g | Sat Fat: 1.8g | Carbohydrates: 18.3g | Fiber: 6.8g | Sugar: 4.3g | Protein: 7.4g

Curried Veggies

Prep Time: 10 minutes
Cook Time: 20 minutes
Serves: 3
Ingredients:
- ½ medium yellow squash, chopped
- ½ medium zucchini, chopped
- ½ onion, thinly sliced
- 1 bell peppers, seeded and cubed
- 1 tablespoon curry powder
- 1 tablespoon olive oil
- Fresh ground black pepper to taste
- 2 tablespoons low-sodium vegetable broth
- 2 tablespoons fresh cilantro, chopped

Preparation:
1. Preheat oven to 375° F and evenly grease large baking dish.
2. Take a bowl and add all the ingredients except cilantro.
3. Now, mix them until well combined.
4. Transfer the vegetable mixture into the prepared baking dish.
5. Bake it for about 15-20 minutes.
6. Serve and enjoy!

Serving Suggestions: Serve it warm with the garnishing of cilantro.
Variation Tip: Add coconut milk for a thicker sauce.
Nutritional Information per Serving:
Calories: 78 | Fat: 5.1g | Sat Fat: 0.7g | Carbohydrates: 8.3g | Fiber: 2.4g | Sugar: 3.9g | Protein: 1.6g

Asparagus Soup

Prep Time: 10 minutes
Cook Time: 40 minutes
Serves: 2
Ingredients:
- ½ tablespoon olive oil
- ¾ pound asparagus, trimmed and chopped
- 1½ scallions, chopped
- 2 cups low-sodium vegetable broth
- 1 tablespoon fresh lemon juice
- ½ Serrano pepper, seeded and chopped finely

Preparation:
1. Take a large frying-pan and heat the oil over medium heat and fry the scallion for about four to five minutes.
2. Stir in the asparagus and broth and bring it to a boil.
3. Reduce the heat to low and let it cook for about 25-30 minutes while covered.
4. Remove the pan from the heat and set aside to let it cool.
5. Now, transfer the soup into a food processor in two batches and pulse until we have a smooth mixture.
6. Transfer the soup into the same pan over medium-heat and cook for about four to five minutes.
7. Stir in the lemon juice, salt and black pepper and remove from the heat.
8. Serve hot.

Serving Suggestions: Serve it with pan-fried or baked salmon to savor the taste.
Variation Tip: You can freeze the soup and can have it later for up to three months.
Nutritional Information per Serving:
Calories: 85 | Fat: 3.8g | Sat Fat: 0.6g | Carbohydrates: 8.7g | Fiber: 4g | Sugar: 3.7g | Protein: 6g

Chicken Lettuce Wraps

Prep Time: 15 minutes
Serves: 1
Ingredients:
- ½ English cucumber, sliced thinly
- ½ tablespoon fresh mint leaves, minced
- 3 ounces cooked chicken breast, cut into strips
- ¼ cup fresh strawberries, hulled and sliced thinly
- 2 large lettuce leaves

Preparation:
1. Take a bowl and add all the given ingredients except for lettuce leaves and gently toss to coat well.
2. Place the lettuce leaves onto serving plates.
3. Divide the chicken mixture over each leaf evenly.
4. Serve immediately.
5. Enjoy!

Serving Suggestions: Serve it with some French fries.
Variation Tip: Place the lettuce into a bowl with ice cubes before using to add a crispy flavor to it.
Nutritional Information per Serving:
Calories: 147 | Fat: 2.6g | Sat Fat: 0.1g | Carbohydrates: 11.8g | Fiber: 2.4g | Sugar: 5.4g | Protein: 19.8g

Roasted Vegetables with Cheese Polenta

Prep Time: 10 minutes
Cook Time: 25 minutes
Servings: 2
Ingredients:
Polenta
- 2 cups low-sodium vegetable or chicken broth
- ½ cup polenta fine cornmeal or corn grits
- ¼ cup goat's cheese
- 1 tablespoon extra-virgin olive oil or butter
- ¼ teaspoon kosher salt
- ¼ teaspoon ground pepper

Vegetables
- 1 tablespoon extra-virgin olive oil or butter
- 1 clove garlic, smashed
- 2 cups roasted root vegetables
- 1 tablespoon torn fresh sage
- 2 teaspoons prepared pesto

Preparation:
1. Place a saucepan over medium heat.
2. Add in the broth and bring it to a boil. Reduce the heat to low.
3. Add in the polenta ingredients and whisk well.
4. Cover the saucepan and cook for 20 minutes, stirring occasionally.
5. After it's done, place the polenta on a serving plate.

6. For the vegetables, take a skillet and place it over medium heat.
7. Add in all the ingredients and cook for 5 minutes while stirring continuously.
8. Put the vegetables on top of the polenta.
9. Serve and enjoy!
Serving Suggestion: Serve with sauce of your choice.
Variation Tip: You can add white pepper to add some more taste.
Nutritional Information per Serving:
Calories: 442|Fat: 27.7g|Sat Fat: 6.7g|Carbohydrates: 41g|Fiber: 7.7g|Sugar: 7.7g|Protein: 9g

Eggplant Parmesan

Prep Time: 15 minutes
Cook Time: 25 minutes
Servings: 6
Ingredients:
• Cooking spray
• 2 eggs
• 2 tablespoons water
• 1 cup panko breadcrumbs
• ¾ cup parmesan cheese, grated and divided
• 1 teaspoon Italian seasoning
• 2 medium eggplants, cut into think slices
• ½ teaspoon salt
• ½ teaspoon ground pepper
• 1 jar tomato sauce
• ¼ cup fresh basil leaves
• 2 cloves garlic, grated
• ½ teaspoon crushed red pepper
• 1 cup mozzarella cheese, shredded
Preparation:
1. Preheat the oven to 400°F.
2. Grease a baking dish with the cooking spray.
3. Whisk the eggs in a bowl.
4. Take another dish and add the Italian seasoning, ¼ cup of parmesan cheese, and the breadcrumbs. Mix well.
5. Place the eggplants on the baking dish and bake for 30 minutes, flipping halfway through. Season with salt and pepper.
6. Take a bowl and add the basil, garlic, pepper, and tomato sauce. Mix well and then place over the eggplant.
7. Top with the seasonings and cheese mixture.
8. Bake for 20–30 minutes.
9. Serve and enjoy!
Serving Suggestion: Serve with basil leaves on top.
Variation Tip: You can skip the red pepper if you want.
Nutritional Information per Serving:

Calories: 241|Fat: 9g|Sat Fat: 4g|Carbohydrates: 28g|Fiber: 6g|Sugar: 9g|Protein: 14g

Quinoa Bowl

Prep Time: 10 minutes
Cook Time: 30 minutes
Servings: 4
Ingredients:
• 1 pound boneless chicken breasts, cooked and sliced
• ¼ teaspoon salt
• ¼ teaspoon ground pepper
• 1 jar roasted red peppers
• ¼ cup slivered almonds
• 4 tablespoons extra-virgin olive oil, divided
• 1 small clove garlic, crushed
• 1 teaspoon paprika
• ½ teaspoon ground cumin
• 2 cups cooked quinoa
• ¼ cup pitted Kalamata olives, chopped
• ¼ cup onion, chopped
• 1 cup cucumber, diced
• ¼ cup feta cheese, crumbled
• 2 tablespoons finely chopped fresh parsley
Preparation:
1. Take a blender and add the garlic, paprika, cumin, peppers, almonds, and 2 tablespoons of oil. Blend until it's in a pureed form.
2. Take a bowl and add the quinoa, onion, olives, and remaining oil. Mix well.
3. Take serving bowls and divide the quinoa mixture evenly between them.
4. Top with the pureed sauce and serve.
Serving Suggestion: Serve with dried basil leaves on top.
Variation Tip: You can add crushed red pepper if you want.
Nutritional Information per Serving:
Calories: 519|Fat: 27g|Sat Fat: 4.5g|Carbohydrates: 31g|Fiber: 4g|Sugar: 2.5g|Protein: 34g

Tortellini Chicken Salad

Prep Time: 10 minutes
Cook Time: 0 minutes
Servings: 6
Ingredients:
- 1 pound chicken breast, cooked (boiled) and sliced
- 2 bay leaves
- 1 package cheese tortellini, boiled
- ½ cup peas
- ¼ cup ranch sauce
- 2 tablespoons red-wine vinegar
- 5 tablespoons basil, chopped
- ½ cup artichokes, divided and chopped
- ½ cup radishes, julienned
- 1 cup peas, boiled
- 2 tablespoons sunflower seeds

Preparation:
1. Take a large bowl and add all the ingredients to it. Mix and toss well to combine.
2. Place into serving bowls.
3. Serve and enjoy!

Serving Suggestion: Serve with basil leaves on top.
Variation Tip: You can also use chia or flax seeds.
Nutritional Information per Serving:
Calories: 357|Fat: 12.7g|Sat Fat: 2.5g|Carbohydrates: 35.5g|Fiber: 4g|Sugar: 3g|Protein: 24g

Shrimp Lemon Pasta

Prep Time: 15 minutes
Cook Time: 15 minutes

Servings: 4
Ingredients:
- 8 ounces whole-wheat fettuccine, boiled
- 1 tablespoon extra-virgin olive oil
- 12 ounces peeled shrimp, cooked
- 2 tablespoons unsalted butter
- 1 tablespoon garlic, finely chopped
- ¼ teaspoon crushed red pepper
- 4 cups loosely packed arugula
- ¼ cup whole-milk plain yogurt
- 1 teaspoon lemon zest
- 2 tablespoons lemon juice
- ¼ teaspoon salt
- $^1/_3$ cup parmesan cheese, grated
- ¼ cup fresh basil, thinly sliced

Preparation:
1. Place a pan over medium heat.
2. Add the garlic and cook for 1 minute. Add in the arugula and cook for 1 more minute.
3. Reduce the heat to low and slowly add the fettuccine, stirring continuously.
4. Add in all the remaining ingredients and mix well.
5. Cook for 5–10 more minutes and serve.

Serving Suggestion: Serve with basil leaves on top.
Variation Tip: You can also top it with parmesan.
Nutritional Information per Serving:
Calories: 403|Fat: 14g|Sat Fat: 6g|Carbohydrates: 45.5g|Fiber: 6g|Sugar: 3g|Protein: 28.3g

Chickpea Quinoa

Prep Time: 10 minutes
Cook Time: 20 minutes
Servings: 4
Ingredients:
- 1 jar roasted red peppers, rinsed
- ¼ cup slivered almonds
- 4 tablespoons extra-virgin olive oil, divided
- 1 clove garlic, minced
- 1 teaspoon paprika
- ½ teaspoon ground cumin
- 2 cups quinoa, cooked
- ¼ cup olives, chopped
- ¼ cup red onion, finely chopped
- 1 can chickpeas, rinsed
- 1 cup cucumber, diced
- ¼ cup feta cheese, crumbled
- 2 tablespoons parsley, chopped

Preparation:

1. Take a blender and add the almonds, peppers, paprika, garlic, cumin, and 2 tablespoons of oil. Blend well until smooth.
2. Take a bowl and add the olives, onion, and quinoa. Mix well.
3. Add the pureed mixture to the olive mixture and combine well.
4. Serve and enjoy!
Serving Suggestion: Serve with cheese on top.
Variation Tip: You can add crushed red pepper if you like.
Nutritional Information per Serving:
Calories: 479|Fat: 25g|Sat Fat: 4.3g|Carbohydrates: 49.5g|Fiber: 7.7g|Sugar: 2.5g|Protein: 12.7g

Roasted Salmon With Chickpeas

Prep Time: 15 minutes
Cook Time: 40 minutes
Servings: 4
Ingredients:
- 2 tablespoons extra-virgin olive oil, divided
- 1 tablespoon smoked paprika
- ½ teaspoon salt, divided, plus a pinch
- 1 can chickpeas, rinsed
- 1/3 cup buttermilk
- ¼ cup mayonnaise
- ¼ cup chives, chopped
- ½ teaspoon ground pepper, divided
- ¼ teaspoon garlic powder
- 10 cups kale, chopped
- ¼ cup water
- 1¼ pounds wild salmon, cut into 4 portions
Preparation:
1. Preheat the oven to 145°F.
2. Take a bowl and add 1 tablespoon of oil, ¼ teaspoon of salt, the paprika, and the chickpeas. Toss well to combine.
3. Take a baking sheet and line it with parchment paper. Add the chickpea mixture and bake for 30 minutes in the preheated oven.
4. Take a food processor and puree the herbs, mayo, buttermilk, ¼ teaspoon of salt, and the garlic powder and set it aside.
5. Take a large skillet and place it over medium heat. Add in the kale and cook it for 2 minutes. Add in the water and cook for 5 more minutes.
6. Now make some space for the salmon in the baking dish and season it with the remaining salt.
7. Bake in the oven for 8 minutes.
8. Place on a serving dish and drizzle the pureed sauce on top.

9. Serve and enjoy!
Serving Suggestion: Serve with a side of veggies.
Variation Tip: You can add some dill for a taste variation.
Nutritional Information per Serving:
Calories: 447|Fat: 21.8g|Sat Fat: 3.7g|Carbohydrates: 23.4g|Fiber: 6.4g|Sugar: 2.2g|Protein: 37g

Tuna Stuffed Avocados

Prep Time: 15 minutes
Serves: 1
Ingredients:
- ½ tablespoon red onion, chopped finely
- 4 tablespoons cooked tuna
- ½ tablespoon fresh cilantro, minced
- ½ large avocado, halved and pitted
- 1 tablespoon fresh lime juice
- Pinch of Cayenne pepper
- Fresh ground black pepper to taste
Preparation:
1. Draw out the flesh from the center of the avocado and transfer into a bowl.
2. Add chopped onion and lemon juice and mash until well combined.
3. Add tuna, cayenne pepper and black pepper and stir to combine everything well.
4. Divide the tuna mixture in both avocado halves evenly.
5. Serve immediately and enjoy!
Serving Suggestions: Serve it with bread and savor the taste.
Variation Tip: Always try to use fresh lime juice instead of bottled ones.
Nutritional Information per Serving:
Calories: 1543 | Fat: 77.2g | Sat Fat: 15.9g | Carbohydrates: 13g | Fiber: 7.1g | Sugar: 1.5g | Protein: 191.1g

Fig and Cheese Salad

Prep Time: 15 minutes
Cook Time: 0 minutes
Servings: 1
Ingredients:
- 2 cups salad greens
- 4 dried figs, stemmed and sliced
- 1 ounce fresh goat's cheese, crumbled
- 1½ tablespoons slivered almonds, preferably toasted
- 2 teaspoons extra-virgin olive oil
- 2 teaspoons balsamic vinegar
- ½ teaspoon honey
- Salt, to taste
- Pepper, to taste

Preparation:
1. Take a large bowl and add all the ingredients.
2. Toss well to combine.
3. Serve and enjoy this yummy salad.

Serving Suggestion: Drizzle some vinegar on top.
Variation Tip: You can add soya sauce for a taste variation.
Nutritional Information per Serving:
Calories: 340|Fat: 21g|Sat Fat: 6g|Carbohydrates: 31.8g|Fiber: 7g|Sugar: 21.8g|Protein: 10.4g

Vegetable Lime Salad

Prep Time: 15 minutes
Cook Time: 30 minutes
Servings: 6
Ingredients:
- ¼ cup canola oil
- ¼ cup extra-virgin olive oil
- 3 tablespoons lime juice
- 1½ tablespoons cilantro, chopped
- ½ teaspoon salt
- ½ teaspoon ground pepper
- 2 cups mixed vegetables, steamed
- 6 lettuce leaves
- 1 small bunch watercress, large stems removed
- 1 large egg, hard-boiled and sliced
- 1 onion, sliced into rings

Preparation:
1. Take a large bowl and add all the ingredients.
2. Toss well to combine.
3. Serve and enjoy this delicious salad!

Serving Suggestion: Serve with cheese on top.
Variation Tip: You can use extra-virgin olive oil instead.
Nutritional Information per Serving:
Calories: 214|Fat: 19.8g|Sat Fat: 2.3g|Carbohydrates: 7.7g|Fiber: 2g|Sugar: 1.8g|Protein: 2.6g

Salmon With Garlic Butter

Prep Time: 15 minutes
Cook Time: 20 minutes
Servings: 4
Ingredients:
- 1 pound salmon fillet, cut into 4 portions
- 1 pound fresh asparagus, trimmed
- ½ teaspoon salt
- ½ teaspoon ground pepper
- 3 tablespoons butter
- 1 tablespoon extra-virgin olive oil
- ½ tablespoon garlic, grated
- 1 teaspoon lemon zest, grated
- 1 tablespoon lemon juice

Preparation:
1. Preheat the oven to 375°F.
2. Grease a baking dish.
3. Place the salmon and asparagus in the baking dish and season them with salt and pepper.
4. Take a skillet, place it over medium heat, add the oil, butter, lemon zest, lemon juice, and garlic and cook until the butter is melted.
5. Drizzle the mixture over the salmon and bake in the preheated oven for 15 minutes.
6. Serve and enjoy.

Serving Suggestion: Serve with potatoes or rice.
Variation Tip: You can also add some white pepper.
Nutritional Information per Serving:
Calories: 270|Fat: 16.5g|Sat Fat: 6.9g|Carbohydrates: 5.6g|Fiber: 2.5g|Sugar: 2.2g|Protein: 25.4g

Garlicky Shrimp

Prep Time: 8 minutes
Cook Time: 7 minutes
Serves: 1
Ingredients:
- 1 garlic clove, minced
- ½ tablespoon fresh cilantro, chopped
- ¼ pound shrimp, peeled and deveined
- ½ tablespoon olive oil
- ½ teaspoon fresh lemon juice
- ½ Serrano pepper, seeded and chopped finely

Preparation:
1. Take a large frying-pan and heat the oil over medium heat and fry garlic and Serrano pepper for about one minute.
2. Include the shrimp and let it cook for about four to five minutes.
3. Stir in lemon juice and remove the pan from the heat.
4. Serve hot with the topping of cilantro.

Serving Suggestions: Serve it with mango salsa for a better taste.
Variation Tip: You can add red pepper flakes to make spicy garlic shrimp.
Nutritional Information per Serving:
Calories: 201 | Fat: 9g | Sat Fat: 1.6g | Carbohydrates: 3g | Fiber: 0.2g | Sugar: 0.2g | Protein: 26.1g

Crusted Salmon

Prep Time: 15 minutes

Cook Time: 10 minutes
Servings: 4
Ingredients:
- 2 teaspoons Dijon mustard
- 1 clove garlic, minced
- ¼ teaspoon lemon zest
- 1 teaspoon lemon juice
- 1 teaspoon rosemary, chopped
- ½ teaspoon honey
- ½ teaspoon kosher salt
- ¼ teaspoon crushed red pepper
- 3 tablespoons panko breadcrumbs
- 3 tablespoons walnuts, finely chopped
- 1 teaspoon extra-virgin olive oil
- 1 pound salmon fillet
- Olive oil cooking spray

Preparation:
1. Preheat the oven to 425°F.
2. Line a baking dish with parchment paper.
3. Add the lemon zest, garlic, mustard, salt, pepper, honey, and rosemary to a mixing bowl. Mix well.
4. Take another bowl and add the panko, oil, and walnuts. Combine well.
5. First, dip the salmon fillets in the mustard sauce and then in the panko mixture.
6. Place the fillets on the lined baking dish.
7. Bake for 12 minutes.
8. Serve and enjoy!

Serving Suggestion: Serve with lemon wedges.
Variation Tip: You can add some parsley leaves while serving too.
Nutritional Information per Serving:
Calories: 222|Fat: 12g|Sat Fat: 2g|Carbohydrates: 4g|Fiber: 1g|Sugar: 2g|Protein: 24g

Chicken and Vegetable Penne Pasta

Prep Time: 15 minutes
Cook Time: 0 minutes
Servings: 4
Ingredients:
- ¾ cup walnuts, chopped
- 1 cup parsley leaves
- 2 cloves garlic, crushed and peeled
- ½ teaspoon plus $1/8$ teaspoon salt
- $1/3$ teaspoon ground pepper
- 2 tablespoons olive oil
- $1/3$ cup parmesan cheese, grated
- 1½ cups chicken breasts, shredded and cooked
- 6 ounces whole-wheat penne pasta, boiled
- 2 cups green beans, boiled
- 2 cups cauliflower florets, boiled

Preparation:
1. Take a small bowl and add walnuts to it. Microwave the bowl for 2 minutes. Set ¼ cup of the walnuts aside.
2. Take a blender and add ½ cup of walnuts, salt, parsley, parmesan, and pepper to it. Blend well until a smooth pesto sauce is formed.
3. Take a bowl and add the pesto sauce and chicken to it. Mix well.
4. Add in the pasta and vegetables. Toss well.
5. Serve and enjoy.

Serving Suggestion: Serve with parsley leaves on top.

Variation Tip: You can add in some oregano for a taste variation.

Nutritional Information per Serving:
Calories: 514|Fat: 26.6g|Sat Fat: 4.2g|Carbohydrates: 43g|Fiber: 9g|Sugar: 4.8g|Protein: 31.4g

Chicken Pasta Salad

Prep Time: 15 minutes
Cook Time: 0 minutes
Servings: 6
Ingredients:
- ½ cup low-fat buttermilk
- ¼ cup low-fat plain Greek yogurt
- 3 tablespoons extra-virgin olive oil
- 2 tablespoons fresh lemon juice
- 2 teaspoons Dijon mustard
- 1½ teaspoons anchovy paste
- 1 large garlic clove
- ¾ cup parmesan cheese, grated and divided
- ½ teaspoon salt, divided
- ½ teaspoon ground pepper, divided
- 8 ounces whole-wheat penne, boiled
- 3 cups chicken breast, cooked and shredded
- 1 pint cherry tomatoes, halved
- 5 cups lettuce, chopped

Preparation:
1. Take a blender and add the buttermilk, oil, yogurt, lemon juice, garlic, anchovy paste, ¼ teaspoon salt, pepper, and ½ cup of parmesan. Blend well until smooth.
2. Take a large bowl and add in the pasta and chicken along with all the remaining ingredients. Mix well.
3. Add in the pureed mixture and toss well to combine.

4. Serve and enjoy!

Serving Suggestion: Serve with cheese on top.
Variation Tip: You can add lime juice for taste variation.

Nutritional Information per Serving:
Calories: 383|Fat: 13.6g|Sat Fat: 3.7g|Carbohydrates: 33.8g|Fiber: 4.4g|Sugar: 4g|Protein: 32.8g

Dijon Salmon

Prep Time: 10 minutes
Cook Time: 12 minutes
Servings: 6
Ingredients:
- 1¼ pounds wild salmon, skinned and cut into 4 portions
- 3 tablespoons extra-virgin olive oil, divided
- 1 tablespoon garlic, minced
- ¾ teaspoon salt
- 2 tablespoons mayonnaise
- 2 teaspoons whole-grain mustard
- ½ teaspoon ground pepper, divided
- 12 ounces green beans, cut into thirds
- 1 lemon zest
- 2 tablespoons pine nuts
- 2 tablespoons water

Preparation:
1. Preheat the oven to 425°F.
2. Line a baking dish with parchment paper.
3. Put the salmon in the prepared baking dish and drizzle it with oil.
4. Add the garlic, salt, mayonnaise, mustard, and ¼ teaspoon of pepper to a blender and blend well. Spread the mixture on top of the salmon.
5. Bake for 8 minutes in the preheated oven.
6. Take a large skillet and place it over medium heat.
7. Add the lemon zest, green beans, pine nuts, and pepper and cook for 4 minutes, stirring occasionally.
8. Serve with the salmon and enjoy.

Serving Suggestion: Serve with rice and veggies.
Variation Tip: You can drizzle some chili sauce on top.

Nutritional Information per Serving:
Calories: 442|Fat: 24.8g|Sat Fat: 3.8g|Carbohydrates: 21.6g|Fiber: 3.8g|Sugar: 1.7g|Protein: 32g

Gnocchi Pomodoro

Prep Time: 35 minutes
Cook Time: 35 minutes
Serves: 4
Ingredients
- 3 tbsp. extra-virgin olive oil, divided
- 1 medium onion, finely chopped
- 2 large cloves garlic, minced
- ¼ tsp. crushed red pepper
- 1½ cups no-salt-added whole tomatoes, pulsed in a food processor until chunky
- ¼ tsp. salt
- 1 tbsp. butter
- ¼ cup chopped fresh basil
- 1 (17.5 oz.) package shelf-stable gnocchi or (12 oz.) package frozen cauliflower gnocchi
- Grated parmesan cheese, for garnish

Preparation
1. Heat 2 tbsp. of the oil in a large skillet over medium heat. Add the onion and cook, stirring, until softened, for about 5 minutes.
2. Add the garlic and crushed red pepper and cook until softened for about 1 minute.
3. Add the tomatoes and salt and bring to a simmer. Reduce the heat to maintain the simmer and cook, stirring often, until thickened (about 20 minutes).
4. Remove from the heat and stir in the butter and basil.
5. Meanwhile, heat the remaining 1 tbsp. of oil in a large non-stick skillet over medium-high heat. Add the gnocchi and cook, stirring often, until plumped and starting to brown (5 to 7 minutes). Add the gnocchi to the tomato sauce and stir until coated.

Serving Suggestion: Serve with tortillas.
Variation Tip: Top with the grated parmesan, if desired.
Nutritional Information Per Serving:
Calories 448 | Protein 10.1g | Carbohydrates 69.4g | Dietary fiber 4.1g | Sugars 5.2g | Fat 14.2g | Sodium 366.6mg

Slow-Cooked Pasta e Fagioli Soup

Prep Time: 8 hours 15 minutes
Cook Time: 15 minutes
Serves: 6
Ingredients
- 2 cups chopped onions
- 1 cup chopped carrots
- 1 cup chopped celery
- 1 lb. pre-cooked chicken thighs, diced
- 4 cups cooked whole-wheat rotini pasta
- 6 cups reduced-sodium chicken broth
- 4 tsp. dried Italian seasoning
- ¼ tsp. salt
- 1 (15 oz.) can no-salt-added white beans, rinsed
- 4 cups baby spinach
- 4 tbsp. chopped fresh basil, divided (optional)
- 2 tbsp. best-quality extra-virgin olive oil
- ½ cup grated Parmigiano-Reggiano cheese

Preparation
1. Place the onions, carrots, and celery in a large sealable plastic bag.
2. Place the cooled, cooked chicken and cooked pasta together in another bag.
3. Seal both bags and freeze for up to 5 days. Defrost the bags in the refrigerator overnight before proceeding.
4. Transfer the vegetable mixture to a large slow cooker. Add the broth, Italian seasoning, and salt. Cover and cook on low for 7¼ hours.
5. Add the beans, spinach, 2 tbsp. of the basil, if using, and the defrosted chicken and pasta. Cook for 45 minutes more. Ladle the soup into bowls.

Serving Suggestion: Serve hot.
Variation Tip: Drizzle a little oil into each bowl and top with cheese and the remaining 2 tbsp. of basil, if desired.
Nutritional Information Per Serving:
Calories 457 | Protein 33.9g | Carbohydrates 42.3g | Dietary fiber 7.6g | Sugars 4.4g | Fat 18.3g | Sodium 653mg

Salmon Couscous Salad

Prep Time: 10 minutes
Cook Time: 10 minutes
Serves: 1
Ingredients
- ¼ cup sliced cremini mushrooms
- ¼ cup diced eggplant
- 3 cups baby spinach
- 2 tbsp. white-wine vinaigrette, divided
- ¼ cup cooked Israeli couscous, preferably whole-wheat
- 4 oz. cooked salmon
- ¼ cup sliced dried apricots
- 2 tbsp. crumbled goat's cheese (½ oz.)

Preparation
1. Coat a small skillet with cooking spray and heat over medium-high heat. Add the mushrooms and eggplant. Cook, stirring, until lightly browned and the juices have been released (3 to 5 minutes). Remove from the heat and set aside.
2. Toss the spinach with 1 tbsp. plus 1 tsp. of vinaigrette and place on a 9-inch plate.

Serving Suggestion: Toss the couscous with the remaining 2 tsp. of vinaigrette and place on top of the spinach. Place the salmon on top. Top with the cooked vegetables, dried apricots, and goat's cheese.
Variation Tip: Add spices of your choice.
Nutritional Information Per Serving:
Calories 464 | Protein 34.8g | Carbohydrates 34.7g | Dietary fiber 5.9g | Sugars 18.9g | Fat 22.1g | Sodium 352.1mg

Cod & Veggies Bake

Prep Time: 10 minutes
Cook Time: 20 minutes
Serves: 2

Ingredients:
- ½ cup zucchini, chopped
- ½ teaspoon olive oil
- 1 tablespoon fresh basil, chopped
- 2½ tablespoons feta cheese, crumbled
- ¼ cup onion, minced
- ½ garlic clove, minced
- 1 cup fresh tomatoes, chopped
- 2 Cod steaks
- Fresh ground black pepper to taste

Preparation:
1. Preheat oven to 450° F.
2. Evenly grease a large shallow baking dish.
3. Take a pan, heat oil over medium heat and fry the onion, zucchini and garlic for about four to five minutes.
4. Stir in the basil, tomatoes, black pepper and immediately remove from the heat.
5. Place the Cod steaks into the prepared baking dish in a single layer and top with tomato mixture evenly.
6. Sprinkle with the cheese evenly.
7. Bake it for about 15 minutes or until they are done.
8. Serve hot.

Serving Suggestions: Serve it with French fries.
Variation Tip: You can tell when the Cod is done if it flakes easily with a fork at the thickest part.
Nutritional Information per Serving:
Calories: 170 | Fat: 6.5g | Sat Fat: 3.7g | Carbohydrates: 12.5g | Fiber: 2.4g | Sugar: 5.1g| Protein: 15.4g

Roasted Salmon With Smoky Chickpeas and Greens

Prep Time: 40 minutes
Cook Time: 40 minutes
Serves: 4
Ingredients
- 2 tbsp. extra-virgin olive oil, divided
- 1 tbsp. smoked paprika
- ½ tsp. salt, divided, plus a pinch
- 1 (15 oz.) can no-salt-added chickpeas, rinsed
- ⅓ cup buttermilk
- ¼ cup mayonnaise
- ¼ cup chopped fresh chives and/or dill, plus more for garnish
- ½ tsp. ground pepper, divided
- ¼ tsp. garlic powder

- 10 cups chopped kale
- ¼ cup water
- 1¼ lbs. wild salmon, cut into 4 portions

Preparation

1. Position racks in the upper third and middle of the oven. Preheat to 425°F.
2. Combine 1 tbsp. of the oil, the paprika, and ¼ tsp. of salt in a medium bowl.
3. Very thoroughly pat the chickpeas dry, then toss with the paprika mixture.
4. Spread the chickpea mixture on a rimmed baking sheet. Bake the chickpeas on the upper rack, stirring twice, for 30 minutes.
5. Meanwhile, puree the buttermilk, mayonnaise, herbs, ¼ tsp. of pepper, and garlic powder in a blender until smooth. Set aside.
6. Heat the remaining 1 tbsp. of oil in a large skillet over medium heat. Add the kale and cook, stirring occasionally, for 2 minutes.
7. Add the water and continue cooking until the kale is tender, about 5 minutes more. Remove from the heat and stir in a pinch of salt.
8. Remove the chickpeas from the oven and push them to one side of the pan. Place the salmon on the other side and season with the remaining ¼ tsp. each of salt and pepper. Bake until the salmon is just cooked through, 5 to 8 minutes.

Serving Suggestion: Drizzle the reserved dressing on the salmon and serve with the kale and chickpeas.
Variation Tip: Garnish with more herbs, if desired.
Nutritional Information Per Serving:
Calories 447 | Protein 37g | Carbohydrates 23.4g | Dietary fiber 6.4g | Sugars 2.2g | Fat 21.8g | Sodium 556.7mg

Prawns & Veggie Curry

Prep Time: 6 minutes
Cook Time: 10 minutes
Serves: 3
Ingredients:
- ½ medium onion
- 1½ garlic cloves, chopped finely
- 1½ medium carrots, peeled and sliced thinly
- ¾ pound prawns, peeled and deveined
- 2 tablespoons water
- 1½ tablespoon fresh basil leaves, chopped
- 1 tablespoon olive oil
- ½ tablespoon fresh ginger, chopped finely
- 1¼ teaspoon curry powder
- ½ cup low-fat sour cream
- 1 medium bell pepper, seeded and sliced
- Fresh ground black pepper to taste

Preparation:

1. Take a large pan, heat the oil over medium-high heat and fry the onion for about four to five minutes.
2. Add ginger, garlic and curry powder and fry them for about a minute.
3. Add bell peppers and carrots and fry them for about three to four minutes.
4. Then, add prawns, sour cream and water and stir them well to combine.
5. Cook for about three to four minutes and stir occasionally.
6. Stir in black pepper and remove from heat.
7. Serve hot and enjoy!

Serving Suggestions: Garnish basil before serving.
Variation Tip: Add some vegetables like beans or cabbage.
Nutritional Information per Serving:
Calories: 298 | Fat: 14.9g | Sat Fat: 6.3g | Carbohydrates: 12.8g | Fiber: 2.1g | Sugar: 4.4g | Protein: 28.2g

Salmon with Salsa

Prep Time: 10 minutes
Cook Time: 8 minutes
Serves: 1
Ingredients:
For Salsa:
- ¼ cup red bell pepper, seeded and chopped
- 1 tablespoon red onion, chopped
- ½ cup fresh pineapple chopped
- ½ tablespoon fresh lemon juice
- Fresh ground black pepper to taste

For Salmon:
- ½ tablespoon extra-virgin olive oil
- 1 tablespoon fresh cilantro leaves, chopped
- 1 Salmon fillets
- Pinch of salt
- Fresh ground black pepper to taste

Preparation:
For Salsa: Take a bowl and mix all the ingredients together.
1. Refrigerate before serving.
For Salmon: First, season salmon with salt and black pepper.
2. In a large frying pan, heat the oil over medium-high heat.
3. Add Salmon, skins side up and cook for about four minutes.
4. Carefully change the side of fillets and cook for about four minutes more.
5. Divide salsa onto both plates alongside salmon fillets and serve.
6. Enjoy!

Serving Suggestions: Serve it lemon on the side and garnish with parsley.
Variation Tip: Cook the salmon until it is flaky on outside and still pink on the inside.
Nutritional Information per Serving:
Calories: 338 | Fat: 18.2g | Sat Fat: 2.6g | Carbohydrates: 10.4g | Fiber: 1.2g | Sugar: 7.1g | Protein: 35.5g

Bruschetta Chicken

Prep Time: 8 minutes
Cook Time: 12 minutes
Serves: 2
Ingredients:
For Chicken:
• 1 chicken boneless, skinless chicken breasts, halved horizontally
• 1½ teaspoon salt-free Italian seasoning
• ½ tablespoon olive oil
• 1 teaspoon garlic, minced
For Topping:
• 1½ garlic cloves, chopped finely
• 2 Roma tomatoes, chopped finely
• 2 tablespoons fresh basil, shredded
• 1 tablespoon olive oil
Preparation:
For Chicken: Take a bowl, add the chicken, garlic and Italian seasoning and mix them well altogether.
1. Take a frying pan and heat the oil over medium-high heat and brown the chicken breasts for about six minutes per side or until done completely.
2. Meanwhile, for Topping: Take a bowl, add all the ingredients except the Parmesan cheese and mix.
3. Remove the frying-pan from the heat and divide the chicken breasts onto serving plates.
4. Serve immediately.
Serving Suggestions: Serve it with crusty bread.
Variation Tip: You can also use fresh tomato cream sauce.
Nutritional Information per Serving:
Calories: 234 | Fat: 13.7g | Sat Fat: 2.6g | Carbohydrates: 5.9g | Fiber: 1.8g | Sugar: 3.5g | Protein: 22.9g

Quinoa Power Salad

Prep Time: 40 minutes
Cook Time: 20 minutes
Serves: 2
Ingredients
• 1 medium sweet potato, peeled and cut into ½-inch thick wedges
• ½ red onion, cut into ¼-inch thick wedges
• 2 tbsp. extra-virgin olive oil, divided
• ½ tsp. garlic powder
• ¼ tsp. salt, divided
• 8 oz. chicken tenders
• 2 tbsp. whole-grain mustard, divided
• 1 tbsp. finely chopped shallot
• 1 tbsp. pure maple syrup
• 1 tbsp. cider vinegar
• 4 cups baby greens, such as spinach, kale, and/or arugula, washed and dried
• ½ cup cooked red quinoa, cooled
• 1 tbsp. unsalted sunflower seeds, toasted
Preparation
1. Preheat the oven to 425°F. Toss the sweet potato and onion with 1 tbsp. of oil, the garlic powder, and ⅛ tsp. of salt in a medium bowl.
2. Spread the mixture on a large rimmed baking sheet and roast for 15 minutes.
3. Meanwhile, add the chicken and 1 tbsp. of the mustard to a bowl. Toss to coat the chicken.
4. When the vegetables have roasted for 15 minutes, remove them from the oven and stir. Add the chicken to the chicken on the baking sheet. Return to the oven and continue roasting until the vegetables start to brown and the chicken is cooked through (about 10 minutes more). Remove from the oven and let cool.
5. Meanwhile, whisk the shallot, maple syrup, vinegar, and the remaining oil, mustard, and salt in a large bowl.
Serving Suggestion: When the chicken has cooled, shred it and place it in the bowl with the dressing. Add the baby greens, quinoa, and the roasted vegetables. Toss with the dressing and sprinkle with sunflower seeds.
Variation Tip: You can prepare the vegetables, chicken, and dressing up to 2 days before serving.
Nutritional Information Per Serving:
Calories 466 | Protein 28.7g | Carbohydrates 35.4g | Dietary fiber 5.5g | Sugars 11.6g | Fat 21.1g | Sodium 716.2mg

84

Slow-Cooked Mediterranean Chicken and Orzo

Prep Time: 4 hours 45 minutes
Cook Time: 15 minutes
Serves: 4
Ingredients
- 1 lb. boneless, skinless chicken breasts, trimmed
- 1 cup low-sodium chicken broth
- 2 medium tomatoes, chopped
- 1 medium onion, halved and sliced
- Zest and juice of 1 lemon
- 1 tsp. herbes de Provence
- ½ tsp. salt
- ½ tsp. ground pepper
- ¾ cup whole-wheat orzo
- ⅓ cup quartered black or green olives
- 2 tbsp. chopped fresh parsley

Preparation
1. Cut the chicken breasts into 4 pieces. Combine the chicken, broth, tomatoes, onion, lemon zest, lemon juice, herbes de Provence, salt, and pepper in a 6-quart slow cooker.
2. Cook on high for 2 hours or on low for 4 hours.
3. Stir in the orzo and olives. Cook for 30 minutes more. Let cool slightly.

Serving Suggestion: Sprinkle with parsley.
Variation Tip: Add spices of your choice.
Nutritional Information Per Serving:
Calories 278 | Protein 29.1g | Carbohydrates 29.5g | Dietary fiber 6.9g | Sugars 3.1g | Fat 4.7g | Sodium 433.8mg

Balsamic Roast Chicken Breast

Prep Time: 10 minutes
Cook Time: 35 minutes
Serves: 2
Ingredients:

- 2, 4 ounces skinless chicken breasts
- black pepper to taste
- 1 teaspoon finely chopped fresh garlic
- 1 tablespoon fresh thyme chopped
- 1 teaspoon grapeseed oil
- ½ cup Balsamic vinegar, plus 2 tablespoons extra
- 8 ounces broccoli florets
- 2 teaspoons Balsamic vinegar
- 2 teaspoons grapeseed oil
- Black pepper to taste
- 2 tablespoons toasted cashew nuts
- Sprigs of fresh parsley to garnish

Preparation:
1. Place the ½ cup Balsamic vinegar, garlic, pepper, thyme and oil in a small pot and bring to a boil.
2. Simmer for about 3 minutes or until the liquid has reduced by about half. Cool this mixture in the freezer for 5 minutes.
3. Oil a baking tray and place the chicken on it. Cover the chicken in the cooled marinade and leave to chill for 30 minutes.
4. Meanwhile, preheat the oven to 375° F. Mix the broccoli florets with two teaspoons of Balsamic vinegar, two teaspoons of grapeseed oil, and pepper.
5. Oil a second baking tray and lay the veg out on it. After 30 minutes, cover the marinated chicken with foil and place in the oven to roast for 30-35 minutes.
6. For the last 15-20 minutes, place the broccoli in the oven to roast too. Give them a good stir at least once while cooking.
7. Once the chicken is cooked, serve it hot with the broccoli on the side.

Serving Suggestion: Garnish with a sprig of parsley, topped with toasted cashews.
Variation Tip: You can swap out the broccoli for Brussel sprouts and use rosemary in the recipe instead of fresh thyme.
Nutritional Information per Serving:
Calories 304 | Fat 12g | Sodium 556mg | Carbs 23g | Fiber 5g | Sugar 8g | Protein 28g

Stuffed Eggplant Shells

Prep Time: 15 minutes
Cook Time: 25 minutes
Serves: 2
Ingredients:
- 1 medium eggplant
- 1 cup water
- 1 tablespoon olive oil
- 4 ounces cooked white beans
- ¼ cup onion, chopped
- ½ cup red, green, or yellow bell peppers, chopped
- 1 cup canned unsalted tomatoes

- ¼ cup tomato liquid
- ¼ cup celery, chopped
- 1 cup fresh mushrooms, sliced
- ¾ cup whole-wheat breadcrumbs
- Black pepper, to taste

Preparation:
1. Preheat the oven to 350°F.
2. Grease a baking dish with cooking spray and set it aside.
3. Trim and cut the eggplant in half, lengthwise.
4. Scoop out the pulp using a spoon and leave the shell about ¼-inch thick.
5. Place the shells in the baking dish with their cut side up.
6. Add water to the bottom of the dish.
7. Dice the eggplant pulp into cubes and set them aside.
8. Add oil to an iron skillet and heat it over medium heat.
9. Stir in the onions, peppers, chopped eggplant pulp, tomatoes, celery, mushrooms, and tomato juice.
10. Cook for 10 minutes on simmering heat, then stir in the beans, black pepper, and breadcrumbs.
11. Divide this mixture into the eggplant shells.
12. Cover the shells with a foil sheet and bake for 15 minutes.
13. Serve warm.

Serving Suggestion: Serve the meal with roasted asparagus on the side.

Variation Tip: Add toasted nuts and seeds on top before serving.

Nutritional Information per Serving:
Calories 305 | Fat 12.7g |Sodium 82mg | Carbs 36g | Fiber 1.4g | Sugar 0.9g | Protein 15.2g

Zucchini Pepper Kebabs

Prep Time: 15 minutes
Cook Time: 40 minutes
Serves: 4
Ingredients:
- 1 small zucchini, sliced into 8 pieces
- 1 red onion, cut into 4 wedges
- 1 green bell pepper, cut into 4 chunks
- 8 cherry tomatoes

- 8 button mushrooms
- 1 red bell pepper, cut into 4 chunks
- ½ cup fat-free Italian dressing,
- ½ cup brown rice
- 1 cup water

Preparation:
1. Toss the tomatoes with the zucchini, onion, peppers, and mushrooms in a bowl.
2. Stir in the Italian dressing and mix well to coat the vegetables.
3. Marinate the mixture for 10 minutes.
4. Bring the water with the rice to a boil in a saucepan, then reduce the heat to a simmer.
5. Cover the rice and cook for 30 minutes until the rice is done.
6. Meanwhile, preheat the broiler on medium heat.
7. Grease the broiler rack with cooking spray and place it 4 inches below the heat source.
8. Put 2 mushrooms, 2 tomatoes, 2 zucchini slices, 1 onion wedge, 1 green pepper slice, and 1 red pepper slice onto a skewer (4 skewers in total).
9. Grill the kebabs for 5 minutes per side.
10. Serve warm.

Serving Suggestion: Serve the meal with boiled rice on the side.

Variation Tip: Add 2 cubes of roasted tofu to each skewer before serving.

Nutritional Information per Serving:
Calories 376 | Fat 11g |Sodium 76mg | Carbs 67g | Fiber 3g | Sugar 4g | Protein 10g

Corn Stuffed Peppers

Prep Time: 15 minutes
Cook Time: 25 minutes
Serves: 4
Ingredients:
- 4 red or green bell peppers
- 1 tablespoon olive oil
- ¼ cup onion, chopped
- 1 green bell pepper, chopped
- 2½ cups fresh corn kernels
- ⅛ teaspoon chili powder
- 2 tablespoons parsley, chopped
- 3 egg whites
- ½ cup skim milk
- ½ cup water

Preparation:

1. Preheat the oven to 350°F.
2. Grease a baking dish with cooking spray.
3. Cut the bell peppers from the top and remove their seeds.
4. Place the peppers in the baking dish with their cut side up.
5. Add the oil to a skillet, then heat it on medium flame.
6. Stir in the onion, corn, and chopped green pepper. Sauté for 5 minutes.
7. Add the cilantro and chili powder. Switch the heat to low.
8. Whisk the milk and egg whites in a bowl.
9. Pour this mixture into the skillet and cook for 5 minutes while stirring.
10. Divide this mixture into each pepper.
11. Add some water to the baking dish.
12. Cover the stuffed peppers with an aluminum sheet.
13. Bake for 15 minutes, then serve warm.

Serving Suggestion: Serve the meal with roasted eggplant on the side.
Variation Tip: Add shredded cheese on top.
Nutritional Information per Serving:
Calories 361 | Fat 16g |Sodium 55mg | Carbs 28g | Fiber 0.1g | Sugar 1.2g | Protein 9g

South Asian Baked salmon

Prep Time: 15 minutes
Cook Time: 20 minutes
Serves: 2
Ingredients:
- ½ cup sugar-free pineapple juice
- 2 garlic cloves, minced
- 1 teaspoon tamari
- ¼ teaspoon ground ginger
- 2 salmon fillets
- ¼ teaspoon sesame oil
- Ground black pepper, to taste
- 1 cup diced fresh fruit, as desired

Preparation:
1. Mix the pineapple juice with the garlic, ginger, and tamari in a bowl.
2. Place the fish in a baking dish.
3. Pour the pineapple mixture over the fish and marinate in the refrigerator for 1 hour, gently flipping the fish halfway through.
4. Meanwhile, preheat the oven to 375°F.

5. Spread out two squares of aluminum foil and layer them with cooking spray.
6. Place the salmon fillets on each square.
7. Top the fish with the sesame oil, pepper, and diced fruit.
8. Fold the aluminum sheets to seal the fish and place them on a baking sheet.
9. Bake for 20 minutes, turning the parcels halfway through.
10. Serve warm.

Serving Suggestion: Serve the fish with roasted broccoli on the side.
Variation Tip: Add crushed red pepper and a drizzle of olive oil on top before serving.
Nutritional Information per Serving:
Calories 245 | Fat 16g |Sodium 131mg | Carbs 12g | Fiber 1.2g | Sugar 4g | Protein 23g

One-Pot Garlicky Shrimp and Spinach

Prep Time: 25 minutes
Cook Time: 25 minutes
Serves: 4
Ingredients
- 3 tbsp. extra-virgin olive oil, divided
- 6 medium cloves garlic, sliced, divided
- 1 lb. spinach
- ¼ tsp. salt plus ⅛ tsp., divided
- 1½ tsp. lemon zest
- 1 tbsp. lemon juice
- 1 lb. shrimp (21–30 count), peeled and deveined
- ¼ tsp. crushed red pepper
- 1 tbsp. finely chopped fresh parsley

Preparation
1. Heat 1 tbsp. of the oil in a large pot over medium heat. Add half the garlic and cook until beginning to brown, 1 to 2 minutes.
2. Add the spinach and ¼ tsp. of the salt and toss to coat. Cook, stirring once or twice until the spinach is mostly wilted, 3 to 5 minutes. Remove from the heat and stir in the lemon juice. Transfer to a bowl and keep warm.
3. Increase the heat to medium-high and add the remaining 2 tbsp. of oil to the pot. Add the remaining garlic and cook until beginning to brown, 1 to 2 minutes.
4. Add the shrimp, crushed red pepper, and the remaining ⅛ tsp. of salt. Cook while stirring until the shrimp are just cooked through, 3 to 5 minutes more.

Serving Suggestion: Serve the shrimp over the spinach, sprinkled with lemon zest and parsley.
Variation Tip: Add more spices, if desired.
Nutritional Information Per Serving:
Calories 226 | Protein 26.4g | Carbohydrates 6.1g | Dietary fiber 2.7g | Sugars 0.7g | Fat 11.6g | Sodium 444mg

Sweet Potato Carbonara With Spinach and Mushrooms

Prep Time: 40 minutes
Cook Time: 20 minutes
Serves: 5
Ingredients
- 2 lbs. sweet potatoes, peeled
- 3 large eggs, beaten
- 1 cup grated parmesan cheese
- ¼ tsp. salt
- ¼ tsp. ground pepper
- 1 tbsp. extra-virgin olive oil
- 3 strips center-cut bacon, chopped
- 8 oz. sliced mushrooms
- 2 cloves garlic, minced
- 5 oz. baby spinach

Preparation
1. Put a large pot of water on to boil.
2. Cut the sweet potatoes lengthwise into long, thin strands using a spiral vegetable slicer or julienne vegetable peeler. You should have about 12 cups of "noodles."
3. Cook the sweet potatoes in the boiling water, gently stirring once or twice, until just starting to soften but not completely tender (around 1½ to 3 minutes). Reserve ¼ cup of the cooking water, then drain. Return the noodles to the pot, off the heat.
4. Combine the eggs, parmesan, salt, pepper, and the reserved water in a bowl. Pour the mixture over the noodles and gently toss with tongs until evenly coated.
5. Heat the oil in a large skillet over medium heat. Add the bacon and mushrooms and cook, stirring often, until the liquid has evaporated and the mushrooms are starting to brown (around 6 to 8 minutes).
6. Add the garlic and cook, stirring, until fragrant, for about 1 minute. Add the spinach and cook, stirring, until wilted, for 1 to 2 minutes. Add the vegetables to the noodles and toss to combine.

Serving Suggestion: Top with a generous grinding of pepper.
Variation Tip: Refrigerate the raw "noodles" for up to 1 day.
Nutritional Information Per Serving:
Calories 312 | Protein 14.5g | Carbohydrates 37.6g | Dietary fiber 5.7g | Sugars 11.6g | Fat 12.2g | Sodium 586.6mg

Hazelnut-Parsley Roast Tilapia

Prep Time: 30 minutes
Cook Time: 20 minutes
Serves: 4
Ingredients
- 2 tbsp. olive oil, divided
- 4 (5 oz.) tilapia fillets (fresh or frozen, thawed)
- ⅓ cup finely chopped hazelnuts
- ¼ cup finely chopped fresh parsley
- 1 small shallot, minced
- 2 tsp. lemon zest
- ⅛ tsp. salt plus ¼ tsp., divided
- ¼ tsp. ground pepper, divided
- 1½ tbsp. lemon juice

Preparation
1. Preheat the oven to 450°F. Line a large rimmed baking sheet with foil and brush with 1 tbsp. of oil.
2. Bring the fish to room temperature by leaving it on the counter for 15 minutes.
3. Meanwhile, stir together the hazelnuts, parsley, shallot, lemon zest, 1 tsp. of oil, ⅛ tsp. salt, and ⅛ tsp. pepper in a small bowl.
4. Pat both sides of the fish dry with a paper towel. Place the fish on the prepared baking sheet. Brush both sides of the fish with lemon juice and the remaining 2 tsp. of oil. Season both sides of the fish evenly with the remaining ¼ tsp. salt and ⅛ tsp. pepper.
5. Divide the hazelnut mixture evenly among the tops of the fillets and pat gently to adhere.
6. Roast the fish until it is opaque, firm, and just beginning to flake (7 to 10 minutes).
Serving Suggestion: Serve immediately.
Variation Tip: Add spices of your choice.
Nutritional Information Per Serving:
Calories 262 | Protein 30.2g | Carbohydrates 3.3g | Dietary fiber 1.2g | Sugars 0.8g | Fat 15g |Sodium 294.7mg.

Fig and Goat's Cheese Salad

Prep Time: 10 minutes
Cook Time: 10 minutes
Serves: 1
Ingredients
- 2 cups mixed salad greens
- 4 dried figs, stemmed and sliced
- 1 oz. fresh goat's cheese, crumbled
- 1½ tbsp. slivered almonds, preferably toasted
- 2 tsp. extra-virgin olive oil
- 2 tsp. balsamic vinegar
- ½ tsp. honey
- Pinch of salt
- Freshly ground pepper to taste

Preparation
1. Combine the greens, figs, goat's cheese, and almonds in a medium bowl.
2. Stir together the oil, vinegar, honey, salt, and pepper.
Serving Suggestion: Just before serving, drizzle the dressing over the salad and toss.
Variation Tip: You can use any other cheese of your choice.
Nutritional Information Per Serving:
Calories 340 | Protein 10.4g | Carbohydrates 31.8g | Dietary fiber 7g | Sugars 21.8g | Fat 21g | Sodium 309.5mg

Masala Chickpeas

Prep Time: 10 minutes
Cook Time: 25 minutes
Serves: 4
Ingredients:
- 1 ½ teaspoon garam masala powder
- 1 teaspoon smoked paprika
- 1 teaspoon jeera powder
- 1 teaspoon ground coriander
- 1 teaspoon turmeric powder
- ¼ teaspoon Cayenne pepper
- 1 tablespoon canola oil
- ½ teaspoon black mustard seeds
- 2 tablespoons jeera seeds 1 white onion, diced
- 4 tablespoons finely chopped garlic
- 1 large sweet red pepper, diced
- 2 rosa tomatoes, roughly chopped
- ½ cup broccoli florets
- 1 medium carrot, peeled and cut into cubes
- 2 cups water
- 30 ounces cooked chickpeas, rinsed and drained
- 1 tablespoon tomato paste
- 10 ounces frozen kale, thawed
- Black pepper to taste
- 2 tablespoons finely chopped fresh coriander, plus extra to garnish

Preparation:
1. In a small bowl, make the spice blend by mixing all the dried spices, except for the jeera seeds and mustard seeds. Set aside.
2. Heat the oil in a medium pot, then add in the mustard seeds and jeera seeds.
3. Cook for 10 seconds before adding in the onion and garlic. Fry for 3 minutes.
4. Add in the following vegetables: red pepper, tomatoes, broccoli, and carrots. Then cook the mixture on medium heat for about 6 minutes.
5. Pour in two cups of water, then add the chickpeas, tomato paste, kale, and black pepper to taste.
6. Bring to a slow boil and cook for about 15-20 minutes, or until the vegetables are cooked through and the stew smells aromatic.
7. Enjoy.
Serving Suggestion: Serve hot, with a sprinkling of freshly chopped coriander.
Variation Tip: You can use any kind of tomato you desire.
Nutritional Information per Serving:
Calories 309 | Fat 7g | Sodium 134mg | Carbs 50g | Fiber 14g | Sugar 17g | Protein 15g

Orecchiette With Broccoli Rabe

Prep Time: 30 minutes
Cook Time: 15 minutes
Serves: 6
Ingredients
- 2 tsp. salt
- 12 oz. orecchiette pasta (about 3½ cups)
- 2 lbs. broccoli rabe (about 2 bunches)
- ¼ cup extra-virgin olive oil
- 3 cloves garlic, chopped
- ½ tsp. crushed red pepper
- 8 anchovy fillets, chopped
- 1 pint cherry tomatoes, halved
Preparation

1. Bring 2 quarts of water to a boil in a large pot. Stir in salt, add the pasta, and cook until just tender. Drain, reserving ½ cup of the water.
2. Meanwhile, thoroughly wash the broccoli rabe and trim off the tough ends. Chop the rabe into 2-inch lengths. Leave some water clinging to the leaves and stems (this will help create a sauce).
3. Heat the oil in a large skillet over medium heat until it starts to shimmer. Add the garlic, crushed red pepper, and anchovies, mashing the fillets until they dissolve.
4. Add the broccoli rabe (you may have to do this in batches, stirring each batch a little until it wilts enough to add more). Cook, stirring, until almost tender (6 to 10 minutes).
5. Add the tomatoes and toss until they begin to soften (about 2 minutes).
6. Add the pasta and toss to coat. If it's too dry, add a little of the reserved pasta water.
Serving Suggestion: Serve immediately.
Variation Tip: Garnish with parmesan if desired
Nutritional Information Per Serving:
Calories 359 | Protein 14.9g | Carbohydrates 49.5g | Dietary fiber 6.9g | Sugars 2.6g | Fat 12.1g | Sodium 388.5mg

3. Seal the bag and shake it to coat well. Refrigerate overnight.
4. Cover the bowl of remaining marinade and refrigerate before serving.
5. Preheat the grill to medium heat.
6. Grease the grill grate finely.
7. Remove the chicken from bag and discard the marinade.
8. Place the chicken onto grill grate and grill it covered for about five to eight minutes per side.
9. Remove chicken from grill and cut into small pieces.
10. Take a large bowl, add the chicken pieces, strawberries and spinach and mix everything together.
11. Place the reserved marinade and toss to coat well.
12. Serve immediately and enjoy!
Serving Suggestions: Serve with lemon juice.
Variation Tip: Try to use fresh strawberries instead of frozen ones.
Nutritional Information per Serving:
Calories: 370 | Fat: 22.9g | Sat Fat: 4.5g | Carbohydrates: 10.8g | Fiber: 2.2g | Sugar: 7.7g | Protein: 34.3g

Chicken & Strawberry Salad

Prep Time: 10 minutes
Cook Time: 16 minutes
Serves: 4
Ingredients:
- 4 tablespoons olive oil
- 1 tablespoon Erythritol
- 2 cups fresh strawberries
- 1 pound boneless, skinless chicken breasts
- 4 tablespoons lemon juice
- ½ garlic clove, minced
- 4 cups fresh spinach, torn
- Pinch of salt
- Fresh ground black pepper to taste
Preparation:
1. For marinade: Take a large bowl and add oil, lemon juice, Erythritol, garlic, salt and black pepper and beat them well until well combined.
2. In a large resalable plastic bag place chicken and ¾ cup marinade.

Mixed Vegetable Salad With Lime Dressing

Prep Time: 30 minutes
Cook Time: 30 minutes
Serves: 6
Ingredients
- ¼ cup canola oil
- ¼ cup extra-virgin olive oil
- 3 tbsp. lime juice
- 1½ tbsp. finely chopped fresh cilantro
- ½ tsp. salt
- ½ tsp. ground pepper
- 2 cups mixed vegetables, steamed (sliced small red potatoes, carrots or beets, green beans, peas) and raw (sliced radishes, cucumbers, or tomatoes)
- 6 leaves romaine or leaf lettuce
- 1 small bunch watercress, large stems removed
- 1 large hard-boiled egg, sliced
- 1 thick slice of red onion, broken into rings
- Crumbled Mexican queso fresco, feta, or farmer cheese for garnish

Preparation
1. Whisk the canola and olive oils, lime juice, cilantro, salt, and pepper in a medium bowl until thoroughly blended. Add the mixed vegetables and toss to coat.
Serving Suggestion: Line a large serving platter with the lettuce. Scoop the dressed vegetables onto the platter. Surround with the watercress and top with the egg, onion, and cheese, if desired.
Variation Tip: Add more spices, if desired.
Nutritional Information Per Serving:
Calories 214 | Protein 2.6g | Carbohydrates 7.7g | Dietary fiber 1.9g | Sugars 1.8g | Fat 19.8g | Sodium 216.6mg

Spinach Ginger Lentils

Prep Time: 10 minutes
Cook Time: 16 minutes
Serves: 4
Ingredients:
- 1 tablespoon olive oil
- 1 shallot, minced
- 1 teaspoon ground ginger
- ½ teaspoon curry powder
- ½ teaspoon ground turmeric
- 1 cup yellow lentils, drained
- 1½ cups vegetable stock
- ½ cup light coconut milk
- 2 cups baby spinach leaves, chopped
- ½ teaspoon salt
Garnish:
- 1 teaspoon white sesame seeds
- 1 tablespoon fresh cilantro, chopped
Preparation:
1. Add the olive oil to a saucepan, then heat it over medium flame.
2. Stir in the ginger, shallot, turmeric, and curry powder.
3. Sauté for 1 minute, then add the stock, coconut milk, and lentils.
4. Let the lentils boil, then reduce the heat to a simmer.
5. Partially cover the pan, then cook for 12 minutes.
6. Meanwhile, toast the sesame seeds in a dry skillet until they turn brown.
7. Add the spinach to the lentils and cook for 3 minutes.
8. Adjust the seasoning with salt.

9. Garnish with the toasted sesame seeds and cilantro.
10. Serve warm.
Serving Suggestion: Serve the meal with roasted cauliflower on the side.
Variation Tip: You can add chopped kale to the lentils as well.
Nutritional Information per Serving:
Calories 263 | Fat 7.5g | Sodium 55mg | Carbs 36g | Fiber 0.4g | Sugar 0.4g | Protein 14g

Coriander-and-Lemon-Crusted Salmon With Asparagus Salad and Poached Egg

Prep Time: 45 minutes
Cook Time: 20 minutes
Serves: 4
Ingredients
- 1 tbsp. coriander seeds
- 1 tsp. lemon zest
- ¾ tsp. fine sea salt, divided
- ½ tsp. crushed red pepper
- 1 lb. wild salmon, skin-on, cut into 4 portions
- 1 lb. asparagus, trimmed
- 2 tbsp. extra-virgin olive oil
- 1 tbsp. lemon juice
- 1 tbsp. chopped fresh mint
- 1 tbsp. chopped fresh tarragon
- ¼ tsp. ground pepper, plus more for garnish
- 8 cups water
- 1 tbsp. white vinegar
- 4 large eggs
Preparation
1. Position a rack in the upper third of the oven and preheat the broiler to high. Coat a rimmed baking sheet with cooking spray.
2. Toast the coriander in a small skillet over medium heat, shaking the pan frequently until fragrant (about 3 minutes).
3. Pulse the coriander, lemon zest, ½ tsp. of salt, and the crushed red pepper in a spice grinder until finely ground.
4. Coat the salmon flesh with the spice mixture (about 1½ tsp. per portion) and place the salmon on the prepared baking sheet.
5. Cut off the asparagus tips and very thinly slice the stalks on the diagonal. Toss the tips and slices with oil, lemon juice, mint, tarragon, pepper, and the remaining salt. Let the mixture stand while you cook the salmon and eggs.

6. Bring the water and vinegar to a boil in a large saucepan.

7. Meanwhile, broil the salmon until just cooked through (3 to 6 minutes), depending on thickness. Tent the salmon with foil to keep it warm.

8. Reduce the boiling water to barely a simmer. Gently stir in a circle, so the water is swirling around the pot. Crack the eggs, one at a time, into the water. Cook until the whites are set, but the yolks are still runny (3 to 4 minutes).

Serving Suggestion: Divide the asparagus salad and salmon among four plates. Make a nest in each salad and top with a poached egg.

Variation Tip: Add more spices of your choice.

Nutritional Information Per Serving:
Calories 288 | Protein 30.5g | Carbohydrates 4.2g | Dietary fiber 1.9g | Sugars 1g | Fat 16.3g | Sodium 360.1mg

Chicken Pesto Pasta With Asparagus

Prep Time: 30 minutes
Cook Time: 15 minutes
Serves: 6
Ingredients
- 8 oz. whole-wheat penne
- 1 lb. fresh asparagus, trimmed and cut into 2-inch pieces
- 3 cups shredded cooked chicken breast
- 1 (7 oz.) container refrigerated basil pesto
- 1 tsp. salt
- ¼ tsp. ground pepper
- 1 oz. parmesan cheese, grated (about ¼ cup)
- Small fresh basil leaves for garnish

Preparation
1. Cook the pasta in a large pot according to package directions.
2. Add the asparagus to the pot during the final 2 minutes of cooking time. Drain, reserving ½ cup of the cooking water.
3. Return the pasta mixture to the pot. Stir in the chicken, pesto, salt, and pepper. Stir in the reserved cooking water 1 tbsp. at a time to reach the desired consistency.

Serving Suggestion: Transfer the mixture to a serving dish. Sprinkle with parmesan and garnish with basil, if desired. Serve immediately.

Variation Tip: Add more spices, if desired.

Nutritional Information Per Serving:
Calories 422 | Protein 31.4g | Carbohydrates 32.2g | Dietary fiber 0.8g | Sugars 3.5g | Fat 18.4g | Sodium 714.1mg

Salmon & Veggie Soup

Prep Time: 10 minutes
Cook Time: 30 minutes
Serves: 2
Ingredients:
- ½ shallot, chopped
- ½ Jalapeno pepper, chopped
- 1 small bell peppers, seeded and chopped
- 1 boneless salmon fillets, cubed
- 1 tablespoon fresh lemon juice
- 1 tablespoon olive oil
- 1 garlic clove, minced
- 2½ cups low-sodium vegetable broth
- ½ head Chinese cabbage, chopped
- 2 tablespoons fresh cilantro, minced
- Fresh ground black pepper to taste

Preparation:
1. Take a large soup pan, heat oil over medium heat and fry shallot and garlic for about two to three minutes.
2. Add cabbage and bell peppers and fry them for about three to four minutes.
3. Add broth and bring to a boil over high heat.
4. Reduce the heat to medium-low and gently cook for about ten minutes.
5. Add salmon and cook for about five to six minutes.
6. Stir in the cilantro, lemon juice and black pepper and cook for about one to two minutes.
7. Serve hot and enjoy!

Serving Suggestions: Serve it with homemade bread.

Variation Tip: You can also vegetables like potatoes and carrots.

Nutritional Information per Serving:
Calories: 250 | Fat: 13.2g | Sat Fat: 1.9g | Carbohydrates: 11.7g | Fiber: 3.1g | Sugar: 5.8g | Protein: 23.8g

Currant Glazed Chops

Prep Time: 15 minutes
Cook Time: 10 minutes
Serves: 6
Ingredients:
- 2 teaspoons olive oil
- 2 tablespoons Dijon mustard
- 6 center-cut pork loin chops
- ¼ cup black currant jam
- ⅓ cup wine vinegar
- ⅛ teaspoon black pepper
- 6 orange slices

Preparation:
1. Mix the jam with the mustard in a bowl.
2. Heat a non-stick skillet, greased with olive oil on medium flame.
3. Place the chops in it and cook for 5 minutes per side.
4. Top the chops with 1 tablespoon of the jam mixture.
5. Cover it and cook for 2 minutes.
6. Transfer the cooked chops to a serving plate.
7. Pour the wine vinegar in the same skillet.
8. Scrape the pork and jam bits from the bottom and sides of the skillet and mix well.
9. Pour the wine mixture over the chops.
10. Season with the pepper and garnish with the orange slices.
11. Serve warm.

Serving Suggestion: Serve the meal with roasted broccoli on the side.
Variation Tip: Add chopped herbs on top.
Nutritional Information per Serving:
Calories 329 | Fat 13g |Sodium 132mg | Carbs 9.1g | Fiber 3g | Sugar 1g | Protein 33g

Salmon and Asparagus With Lemon-Garlic Butter Sauce

Prep Time: 25 minutes
Cook Time: 10 minutes
Serves: 4
Ingredients

- 1 lb. center cut salmon fillet, preferably wild, cut into 4 portions
- 1 lb. fresh asparagus, trimmed
- ½ tsp. salt
- ½ tsp. ground pepper
- 3 tbsp. butter
- 1 tbsp. extra-virgin olive oil
- ½ tbsp. grated garlic
- 1 tsp. grated lemon zest
- 1 tbsp. lemon juice

Preparation
1. Preheat the oven to 375°F. Coat a large rimmed baking sheet with cooking spray.
2. Place the salmon on one side of the prepared baking sheet and the asparagus on the other. Sprinkle the salmon and asparagus with salt and pepper.
3. Heat the butter, oil, garlic, lemon zest, and lemon juice in a small skillet over medium heat until the butter is melted. Drizzle the butter mixture over the salmon and asparagus.
4. Bake until the salmon is cooked through and the asparagus is just tender, 12 to 15 minutes.

Serving Suggestion: Serve hot with tortillas.
Variation Tip: Add spices of your choice.
Nutritional Information Per Serving:
Calories 270 | Protein 25.4g | Carbohydrates 5.6g | Dietary fiber 2.5g | Sugars 2.2g | Fat 16.5g | Sodium 350.5mg

Pork with Herbs de Provence

Prep Time: 10 minutes
Cook Time: 6 minutes
Serves: 2
Ingredients:
- 8 ounces pork tenderloin
- Black pepper, to taste
- ½ teaspoon herbs de Provence
- ¼ cup dry white wine

Preparation:
1. Season the pork tenderloin with the black pepper.
2. Place the pork on parchment paper and pound it with a mallet to get a ¼-inch thick piece.
3. Heat a non-stick wok or frying pan and add the pork to it.
4. Cook for 3 minutes per side until brown.
5. Sprinkle the herbs de Provence on top.
6. Transfer the pork to a serving plate.

7. Add the wine to the same pan and cook until it boils.
8. Pour it over the pork and serve warm
Serving Suggestion: Serve the pork with roasted potatoes on the side.
Variation Tip: Add chopped herbs on top.
Nutritional Information per Serving:
Calories 250 | Fat 7.9g |Sodium 81mg | Carbs 4g | Fiber 2.6g | Sugar 0.1g | Protein 25g

Seafood Stew

Prep Time: 10 minutes
Cook Time: 30 minutes
Serves: 4
Ingredients:
- ½ medium yellow onion, chopped
- ½ Jalapeno pepper, chopped
- ½ pound red snapper fillets, cubed
- ¼ pound fresh tomatoes, chopped
- ⅛ pound fresh squid, cleaned and cut into rings
- ⅛ pound mussels
- ¼ cup fresh parsley, chopped
- 1 tablespoon olive oil
- 3/2 garlic cloves, minced
- ⅛ teaspoon red pepper flakes, crushed
- ¾ cup low-sodium fish broth
- ¼ pound shrimp, peeled and deveined
- ⅛ pound bay scallops
- 1 tablespoon fresh lemon juice

Preparation:
1. Take a large soup pan, heat oil over medium heat and fry the onion for about five to six minutes.
2. Add the garlic, Serrano pepper and red pepper flakes and fry for another minute.
3. Include tomatoes and broth and bring to a gentle simmer.
4. Reduce the heat to low and cook for about ten minutes.
5. Add the snapper and cook for about two minutes.
6. Stir in the remaining seafood and cook for about six to eight minutes.
7. Stir in the lemon juice, basil, salt and black pepper and remove from heat.
8. Serve hot and enjoy!
Serving Suggestions: Garnish with freshly chopped herbs or bacon crumbles.
Variation Tip: You can also use mussels and white fish.
Nutritional Information per Serving:
Calories: 1024 | Fat: 18.6g | Sat Fat: 4.4g | Carbohydrates: 33g | Fiber: 1.1g | Sugar: 1.7g | Protein: 168.7g

Herbed White Sea Bass

Prep Time: 10 minutes
Cook Time: 10 minutes
Serves: 2
Ingredients:
- 2 white sea bass fillets, each 4 ounces
- 1 tablespoon lemon juice
- 1 teaspoon garlic, minced
- ¼ teaspoon herb seasoning blend
- Ground black pepper, to taste
Preparation:
1. Preheat the broiler and place its rack about 4 inches below the heat source.
2. Grease a baking pan with cooking spray.
3. Place the fish fillets in the baking pan.
4. Add the lemon juice, pepper, herbed seasoning, and garlic on top of the fish.
5. Place the baking pan in the broiler.
6. Cook for 10 minutes.
7. Serve warm.
Serving Suggestion: Serve the meal with roasted carrots on the side.
Variation Tip: Add crushed red pepper on top before serving.
Nutritional Information per Serving:
Calories 125 | Fat 14g |Sodium 141mg | Carbs 1g | Fiber 0.3g | Sugar 1g | Protein 21g

Chipotle Tomato Shrimp

Prep Time: 10 minutes
Cook Time: 8 minutes
Serves: 4
Ingredients:
- ¾ pound uncooked shrimp, peeled and deveined
- 2 tablespoons tomato paste
- 1½ teaspoons water

- ½ teaspoon olive oil
- ½ teaspoon minced garlic
- ½ teaspoon chipotle chili powder
- ½ teaspoon fresh oregano, chopped

Preparation:
1. Rinse and dry the shrimp and set it aside.
2. Mix the tomato paste with the water, oil, chili powder, oregano, and garlic in a bowl.
3. Spread the marinade over the shrimp using a brush.
4. Coat well on both sides of the shrimp.
5. Marinate the shrimp in the refrigerator until the broiler is ready.
6. Preheat the broiler on medium heat.
7. Grease the broiler rack with oil and place it 6 inches below the heat source.
8. Thread the shrimp onto skewers and grill them for 4 minutes per side.
9. Serve warm.

Serving Suggestion: Serve the prawns with roasted cauliflower on the side.

Variation Tip: Add sesame seeds or chopped herbs on top.

Nutritional Information per Serving:
Calories 185 | Fat 16g |Sodium 62mg | Carbs 13g | Fiber 0.4g | Sugar 3g | Protein 33g

Shrimp Ceviche

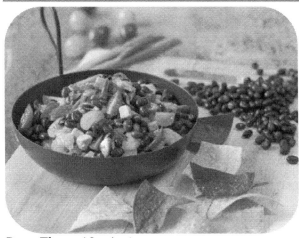

Prep Time: 10 minutes
Cook Time: 10 minutes
Serves: 4
Ingredients:
- ½ pound raw shrimp
- 2 lemons, zest and juice
- 2 limes, zest and juice
- 2 tablespoons olive oil
- 2 teaspoons cumin
- ½ cup red onion, diced
- 1 cup tomato, diced
- 2 tablespoons garlic, minced
- 1 cup black beans, cooked
- ¼ cup serrano chili pepper, diced and seeds removed
- 1 cup cucumber, peeled and diced
- ¼ cup cilantro, chopped

Preparation:
1. Spread the shrimp in a shallow dish and drizzle the lime and lemon juice over the top.
2. Refrigerate the shrimp for 3 hours to make the ceviche.
3. Combine the remaining ingredients and set them aside.
4. Add the shrimp to this mixture.
5. Serve with tortilla chips.

Serving Suggestion: Serve the meal with roasted green beans on the side.

Variation Tip: Add crushed nuts or chopped cranberries to the ceviche.

Nutritional Information per Serving:
Calories 305 | Fat 25g |Sodium 132mg | Carbs 13g | Fiber 0.4g | Sugar 2g | Protein 28.3g

Spinach and Zucchini Risotto

Prep Time: 10 minutes
Cook Time: 40 minutes
Serves: 4
Ingredients:
- 8 cups chicken broth
- 10 ounces zucchini, diced
- 1 cup wild rice
- 10 ounces spinach, trimmed and finely sliced
- 2 tablespoons olive oil
- 4 garlic cloves, crushed
- Zest and juice of 1 lemon
- ¼ chopped fresh thyme
- 1 cup white wine

Preparation:
1. Bring the broth just to a simmer in a large pot.
2. Heat the olive oil in a large skillet over medium heat for 30 to 60 seconds until it begins to shimmer. Put in the garlic and cook for 30 seconds.
3. Add the rice. Cook, often stirring, for about 1 minute, and then pour in the wine. Continue to stir and cook until the wine thoroughly combines with the rice.
4. Spread the lemon zest and pour in juice, and stir.
5. Reduce the heat to medium-low, and spring about 1 cup of the warm broth with a ladle into the skillet.
6. Cook, often stirring, until the liquid combines with the mixture thoroughly.
7. Pour in another cup of broth and continue stirring once again until the liquid combines thoroughly with the mixture.
8. Repeat with additional broth until the rice is creamy and cooked through for a thick consistency.
9. Remove the skillet from the heat and add the zucchini and thyme.
10. Serve warm.

Serving Suggestion: Garnish with basil leaves.

Variation Tip: If you want to make a more traditional risotto, add 1 to 2 tablespoons of margarine and ½ to ¾ cup of finely grated, low-fat Parmigiano-Reggiano cheese right before you add the asparagus.

Nutritional Information per Serving:
Calories 288 | Fat 7g | Sodium 6mg | Carbs 42g | Fiber 3g | Sugar 0g | Protein 6g

Chicken Tikka

Prep Time: 10 minutes
Cook Time: 8 minutes
Serves: 6
Ingredients:
- 4 chicken breasts, skinless, boneless; cubed
- 2 large onions, cubed
- 10 cherry tomatoes
- ⅓ cup plain non-fat yogurt
- 4 garlic cloves, crushed
- 1 ½ inch fresh ginger, peeled and chopped
- 1 small onion, grated
- 1 ½ teaspoon chili powder
- 1 tablespoon ground coriander
- 1 teaspoon salt
- 2 tablespoons of coriander leaves

Preparation:
1. Combine the non-fat yogurt, crushed garlic, ginger, chili powder, coriander, salt and pepper in a large bowl.
2. Add the cubed chicken; stir until the chicken is coated. Cover with plastic film, place in the fridge. Marinate 2-4 hours. Heat the barbecue.
3. After marinating the chicken, get some skewers ready.
4. Alternate pieces of chicken cubes, cherry tomatoes and cubed onions onto the skewers.
5. Grill for 6-8 minutes on each side.
6. Once the chicken is cooked through, pull the meat and vegetables off the skewers onto plates.
7. Serve immediately.
Serving Suggestion: Garnish with coriander.
Variation Tip: For a milder taste, omit the chili powder.
Nutritional Information per Serving:
Calories 117 | Fat 19 g | Sodium 203 mg | Carbs 59 g | Fiber 0.3g | Sugar 0.5 g | Protein 19 g

Pumpkin Rice

Prep Time: 10 minutes
Cook Time: 15 minutes
Serves: 4
Ingredients:
- 12 ounces sliced pumpkins
- 1 cup dry instant brown rice

- 3 scallion stalks, thinly sliced and separated
- 2 teaspoons olive oil
- 1 teaspoon dried rosemary
- 1 teaspoon ground allspice
- 2 cups water
- 2 cups white beans, frozen
- ¼ cup shredded homemade mozzarella cheese

Preparation:
1. Heat the olive oil in a large saucepan over medium-high heat.
2. Add the pumpkins, the white parts of the scallions, and the ground allspice and sauté until the pumpkins are just cooked through about 5 minutes.
3. Add water and rosemary and boil over high heat.
4. Whisk in the rice, white beans and half of the green parts of the scallions.
5. Bring the heat to medium and cook, stirring from time to time, for 7 minutes, or until the rice is warm and the white beans are softened.
6. Smear each serving with cheese and the reserving green parts of the scallions.
7. Serve warm.
Serving Suggestion: Garnish with thyme sprigs.
Variation Tip: You can use any type of mushrooms you like in this recipe.
Nutritional Information per Serving:
Calories 220 | Fat 4g | Sodium 11mg | Carbs 40g | Fiber 9g | Sugar 1g | Protein 10g

Poached Salmon with Mustard-Dill Sauce

Prep Time: 10 minutes
Cook Time: 15 minutes
Serves: 2
Ingredients:
- 1½ teaspoons cornstarch
- 1 tablespoon lemon juice
- Black pepper to taste
- 2 teaspoons Dijon mustard
- 1 teaspoon olive oil
- 2 tablespoons fresh dill, chopped
- ¼ cup reduced-fat sour cream
- 1¼ pound salmon fillet, cut into 4 portions
- 2 tablespoons shallots, finely chopped
- 1½ cup fat-free milk
- ½ teaspoon salt

Preparation:
1. Preheat the oil in a 10-inch skillet over medium heat.
2. Add the shallots and sauté for 1 minute.
3. Stir in the milk, salt, and pepper. Bring the mixture to a simmer.

4. Add the salmon pieces and cook for 10 to 12 minutes.
5. Transfer the fish to a plate using a slotted spoon.
6. Cover the fish with foil and set it aside.
7. Mix the lemon juice with the cornstarch in a bowl.
8. Pour this slurry into the skillet and cook for 1 minute.
9. Stir in the dill, mustard, and sour cream.
10. Pour this sauce over the cooked fish.
11. Serve warm.
Serving Suggestion: Serve with fresh sautéed vegetables of your choice.
Variation Tip: Add a sprinkle of herbs on top.
Nutritional Information per Serving:
Calories 301 | Fat 15g |Sodium 40mg | Carbs 17g | Fiber 1.2g | Sugar 1.3g | Protein 28.3g

Healthy Mac and Cheese

Prep Time: 10 minutes
Cook Time: 25 minutes
Serves: 4
Ingredients:
• 8 ounces 100% whole wheat macaroni pasta
• 1/3 cup low-fat Ricotta cheese, divided
• 1 cup shredded low-fat Cheddar cheese, divided
• ½ cup whole wheat bread crumbs
• ½ cup grated Parmesan cheese
• ½ cup water
• 1 large white onion, sliced
• 8 medium cloves garlic, halved
• ⅛ teaspoon Sea salt
• ⅛ teaspoon cracked black pepper
• 1 teaspoon brown mustard
• 1 cup coarsely chopped broccoli florets
• Pinch of chili pepper flakes
• ¼ teaspoon dried basil
• 1 tablespoon chopped fresh parsley
Preparation:
1. Preheat the oven to 425° F.
2. Coat a 9-9-inch baking dish with olive oil spray and set aside.
3. Add the water, onion, and garlic to a medium saucepan. Cover with a lid and simmer over low heat for about 10 minutes, or until onion and garlic can easily be mashed with a fork.
4. Put the mixture into a blender, add salt, pepper, mustard and pulse to combine.
5. Bring a large pot of water to boil, add the pasta and cook according to package directions until al dente. In the last few minutes of boiling the pasta, add the broccoli and cover the pot.
6. After about 3 minutes, drain the pasta and broccoli and run under cold water so that the pasta does not keep cooking.

7. Heat the pasta pot over low heat, and add the onion-garlic paste, chili pepper flakes and two tablespoons of the Ricotta.
8. Stir until the cheese is incorporated, and then slowly stir in the rest of the Ricotta with a whisk.
9. Add half of the Cheddar cheese, and stir until melted. Then add the rest of the Cheddar cheese, and stir until melted.
10. Add the cooked pasta and broccoli, and stir with a large spoon until the sauce covers most of the pasta.
11. Top with bread crumbs, Parmesan cheese and basil.
12. Bake for about 10 minutes, or until the bread crumbs and Parmesan start to brown.
13. Remove from the oven, and serve warm.
Serving Suggestion: Top with parsley.
Variation Tip: Substitute macaroni with whole wheat Rotini pasta or whole wheat penne pasta. Use just about any veggies, such as cauliflower, zucchini, bell peppers and spinach. Low-fat Cottage cheese can be used in place of Ricotta cheese.
Nutritional Information per Serving:
Calories 366 | Fat 9 g | Sodium 511 mg | Carbs 44 g | Fiber 8 g | Sugar 0.7 g | Protein 25 g

Asparagus Cheese Vermicelli

Prep Time: 15 minutes
Cook Time: 10 minutes
Serves: 3
Ingredients:
• 2 teaspoons olive oil, divided
• 6 asparagus spears, cut into pieces
• 4 ounces dried whole-grain vermicelli
• 1 medium tomato, chopped
• 1 tablespoon garlic, minced
• 2 tablespoons fresh basil, chopped
• 4 tablespoons parmesan, freshly grated, divided
• 1/8 teaspoon black pepper, ground
Preparation:
1. Add 1 teaspoon of oil to a skillet and heat it.
2. Stir in the asparagus and sauté until golden brown.
3. Cut the sautéed asparagus into 1-inch pieces.
4. Fill a pot with water up to ¾ full and bring to a boil.
5. Add the pasta and cook for 10 minutes or until it is done.
6. Drain and rinse the pasta under running water.
7. Add the pasta to a large bowl, then toss in the olive oil, tomato, garlic, asparagus, basil, garlic, and parmesan.
8. Serve with black pepper on top.
9. Enjoy.

Serving Suggestion: Serve the meal with roasted mushrooms on the side.
Variation Tip: Add crushed red pepper on top before serving.
Nutritional Information per Serving:
Calories 325 | Fat 8g |Sodium 50mg | Carbs 48g | Fiber 1g | Sugar 1.2g | Protein 2g

Chicken & Broccoli Casserole

Prep Time: 10 minutes
Cook Time: 45 minutes
Serves: 3
Ingredients:
- 1½ broccoli heads, cut into florets
- 2 tablespoons extra-virgin olive oil
- 2 garlic cloves, minced
- 3 skinless, boneless chicken thighs
- ½ teaspoon dried rosemary, crushed
- ½ teaspoon dried oregano, crushed
- Fresh ground black pepper to taste

Preparation:
1. Preheat oven to 375° F and evenly grease a large baking dish.
2. Take a large bowl and add all the ingredients and toss to coat well.
3. Now, in the bottom of the dish arrange the broccoli florets and top it with chicken breasts in a single layer.
4. Bake it for about 45 minutes.
5. Serve hot and enjoy!
Serving Suggestions: Serve it with crackers or bread crumbs as a topping.
Variation Tip: You can also add pre-cooked chicken.
Nutritional Information per Serving:
Calories: 240 | Fat: 13.6g | Sat Fat: 2.9g | Carbohydrates: 4g | Fiber: 1.4g | Sugar: 0.8g | Protein: 26.4g

Spicy Seafood Stew

Prep Time: 10 minutes
Cook Time: 25 minutes
Serves: 4
Ingredients:
- 8 ounces fresh skinless fish fillets, cut into pieces
- 6 ounces fresh shrimp, peeled and deveined
- 2 teaspoon olive oil

- ⅔ cup chopped onion
- ½ cup finely chopped carrot
- ½ cup red pepper, chopped
- 2 cloves garlic, minced
- 1 14-½-ounce can low-sodium tomatoes, undrained and cut up
- 1 8 ounces can of low-sodium tomato sauce
- 1 cup reduced-sodium chicken broth
- ¼ cup red wine
- 2 bay leaves
- 1 tablespoon snipped fresh thyme
- ½ teaspoon Cajun seasoning
- ¼ teaspoon ground cumin
- ¼ teaspoon crushed red pepper

Preparation:
1. Heat 2 teaspoon oil in a cooking pot and add onion, garlic, carrot and sweet pepper.
2. Sauté for 5 minutes, add tomato sauce, broth, wine, tomatoes, bay leaves, dried thyme, cumin, red pepper and Cajun seasoning.
3. Bring Cajun mixture to a boil and cook for 20 minutes at a low simmer.
4. Add fresh thyme and seafood. Cover the lid and cook for 5 minutes.
5. Serve warm.
Serving Suggestion: Garnish with parsley.
Variation Tip: Feel free to use any kind of filleted fish.
Nutritional Information per Serving:
Calories 298 | Fat 5.7 g | Sodium 394 mg | Carbs 12.4 g | Fiber 0.2g | Sugar 0 g | Protein 16.9 g

Mixed Vegetarian Chili

Prep Time: 15 minutes
Cook Time: 36 minutes
Serves: 4
Ingredients:
- 1 tablespoon olive oil
- 14 ounces canned black beans, drained
- ½ cup yellow onion, chopped
- 12 ounces extra-firm tofu, cut into pieces
- 14 ounces canned kidney beans, drained
- 2 cans (14 ounces each) diced tomatoes
- 3 tablespoons chili powder
- 1 tablespoon oregano
- 1 tablespoon cilantro, chopped
Preparation:

1. Take a soup pot and heat olive oil in it over medium heat.
2. Add the onions and sauté for 6 minutes until soft.
3. Add the tomatoes, beans, chili powder, oregano, and beans.
4. Bring to a boil, then reduce the heat to a simmer.
5. Cook for 30 minutes, then add the cilantro.
6. Serve warm.
Serving Suggestion: Serve the meal with roasted tortillas on the side.
Variation Tip: Add avocado slices and roasted broccoli on top before serving.
Nutritional Information per Serving:
Calories 391 | Fat 5g |Sodium 88mg | Carbs 43g | Fiber 0g | Sugar 0g | Protein 19g

Chicken and Broccoli Stir-Fry

Prep Time: 10 minutes
Cook Time: 15 minutes
Serves: 4
Ingredients:
• 2 boneless, skinless chicken breasts, cubed
• 2 tablespoons olive oil, divided
• 3 small carrots, thinly sliced
• 15 ounces frozen chopped broccoli florets, thawed
• 8 ounces sliced water chestnuts, drained and thoroughly rinsed
• 2 garlic cloves, minced
• 2 teaspoons ground ginger
• 3 tablespoons Balsamic vinegar, divided
Preparation:
1. In a wok or large sauté pan, add ½ tablespoon olive oil and heat over medium heat.
2. Place the cubed chicken and fried about 5 to 7 minutes, until lightly browned and cooked through.
3. Remove chicken from the pan to a bowl with a lid and set aside.
4. Pour the olive oil, garlic, and carrots into the pan and heat over medium heat until the carrots soften, about 3 to 4 minutes.
5. Place the thawed broccoli florets, water chestnuts and Balsamic vinegar into it and cook another for 3 to 4 minutes.
6. Mix the cooked chicken with 2 tablespoons Balsamic vinegar and two teaspoons of ground ginger and stir until well coated.
7. Enjoy.
Serving Suggestion: Serve over brown rice if you want.
Variation Tip: Add some hot sauce, whose heat can mask the missing salty flavor.
Nutritional Information per Serving:
Calories 189 | Fat 9g | Sodium 68mg | Carbs 12g | Fiber 3g | Sugar 3g | Protein 14g

Turkey Burger

Prep Time: 10 minutes
Cook Time: 10 minutes
Serves: 4
Ingredients:
• Nonstick cooking spray
• 2 tablespoons extra-virgin olive oil (if not grilling)
• 1 pound ground turkey
• Roasted carrots and beets
• 4 (1-ounce) low-fat Cheddar cheese slices
• 4 whole-wheat hamburger buns
• ¼ teaspoon salt
• ¼ teaspoon freshly ground black pepper
• 2 tablespoons wholegrain mustard
• 1 cup chopped kale leaves
• 1 medium tomato, sliced
• ½ medium red onion, sliced
Preparation:
1. Roast the carrots and beets. Coat the grill grates with cooking spray. Preheat the grill to high heat. (Alternatively, heat the oil in a skillet over medium-high heat.) Form the turkey into four equal patties and season with salt and pepper.
2. Grill the patties covered for 5 minutes. Flip and continue to cook covered for an additional 5 minutes. (Same time if cooking in a skillet.)
3. Place a patty and a slice of Cheddar cheese in each of 4 storage containers. Store the buns, mustard, kale, tomato, onion, roasted carrots and beets separately.
4. When ready to serve, reheat the patties for 1 minute.
5. Top with the cheese and heat together long enough for the cheese to melt. Split and toast the buns.
6. Spread the toasted buns with mustard and assemble the burgers with kale, tomato, and onion.
7. Enjoy.
Serving Suggestion: Serve with the roasted vegetables.
Variation Tip: If you don't have whole grain mustard at home, top with ketchup, mayonnaise or sliced avocado instead.
Nutritional Information per Serving:
Calories 690 | Fat 41g | Sodium 910mg | Carbs 46g | Fiber 9.5g | Sugar 24g | Protein 32g

Turkey Stir Fry with Vegetables

Prep Time: 10 minutes
Cook Time: 30 minutes
Serves: 2
Ingredients:
- 1 cup turkey, cooked, cut into ½-inch cubes
- 2 cups vegetables
- 2 cups brown rice, cooked
- 1 tablespoon oil
- ½ teaspoon sugar
- ½ tablespoon ginger, minced
- ¼ teaspoon clove garlic, minced
- ½ teaspoon salt

Preparation:
1. In a nonstick frying pan, heat oil at low-medium temperature. Put the turkey, vegetables, minced ginger, garlic and salt.
2. Stir and fry for about one minute.
3. Add sugar and continue stirring. Reduce heat to avoid scorching and continue cooking until the vegetables become tender.
4. When the vegetables become tender, remove them from the heat.
5. If the vegetables do not cook well, pour 2-3 tablespoons of water and cook until soft.
Serving Suggestion: Serve with the cooked rice.
Variation Tip: Feel free to use fresh or frozen, or canned vegetables.
Nutritional Information per Serving:
Calories 223 | Fat 12g | Sodium 598mg | Carbs 21g | Fiber 6g | Sugar 8g | Protein 13g

Grouper Curry

Prep Time: 15 minutes
Cook Time: 15 minutes
Serves: 10

Ingredients:
- 4 tablespoons fresh basil leaves, chopped

- 2½ cups unsweetened coconut milk
- 3 tablespoons salt-free curry paste
- 2 teaspoons fresh ginger, minced
- 2 small yellow onion, chopped
- 2 tablespoons olive oil
- 4 garlic cloves, minced
- 2 large tomato, peeled and chopped
- ½ cup water
- 3 pounds skinless grouper fillets, cubed
Preparation:
1. Grab a large frying-pan and heat the oil over medium heat and fry the onion, garlic and ginger for about five minutes.
2. Include the tomatoes and cook for about two to three minutes, crushing with the back of the spoon.
3. Add the curry paste and fry for another two minutes.
4. Add the water and coconut milk and bring to a gentle boil.
5. Stir in grouper pieces and cook for about four to five minutes.
6. Stir in the basil leaves.
7. Serve hot and enjoy!
Serving Suggestions: Serve with dried curry leaves.
Variation Tip: You can use a hot curry powder if you prefer a little spice.
Nutritional Information per Serving:
Calories: 383 | Fat: 20.5g | Sat Fat: 13.5g | Carbohydrates: 12.7g | Fiber: 3.7g | Sugar: 4.8g | Protein: 37.9g

Tofu Stir-Fry

Prep Time: 10 minutes
Cook Time: 15 minutes
Serves: 4
Ingredients:
- 1 tablespoon canola oil
- 2 large garlic cloves, minced
- 2½ tablespoons reduced-sodium soy sauce, divided
- 1 tablespoon minced fresh ginger
- 1 small bunch of scallions, finely chopped, divided
- 1 cup sugar snap peas
- 1 cup small broccoli florets
- ½ cup diced carrots
- ½ cup sliced red bell pepper
- 1 tablespoon honey
- 10 ounces spinach leaves, divided
- 2 (14 ounces) packages extra-firm tofu, drained, patted dry and cut into ¾-inch cubes
Preparation:
1. In a large wok, sauté pan, or deep skillet, heat the oil over medium heat and swirl to coat the entire pan.
2. Once hot, add the garlic, one tablespoon of soy sauce and ginger. Stir well for about a minute.
3. Add the scallions, snap peas, broccoli, carrots and bell pepper and stir-fry for 5 to 8 minutes, or until the vegetables are crisp-tender.
4. Add the remaining 1½ tablespoons of soy sauce and honey. Add 5 ounces of spinach, making sure to stir as it cooks down.

5. Once it has wilted, add the remaining 5 ounces of spinach.
6. Stir until it has cooked down.
7. Add the tofu and continue occasionally stirring for 2 to 3 minutes to give the tofu time to absorb the flavors.
Serving Suggestion: Top with chopped parsley.
Variation Tip: For a vegan option: Use agave instead of honey.
Nutritional Information per Serving:
Calories 304 | Fat 14g | Sodium 445mg | Carbs 21g | Fiber 7g | Sugar 4.7g | Protein 25g

Southwestern Vegetable Tacos

Prep Time: 15 minutes
Cook Time: 11 minutes
Serves: 8
Ingredients:
- 1 tablespoon olive oil
- 1 cup red onion, chopped
- 1 cup yellow squash, diced
- 1 cup green zucchini, diced
- 3 large garlic cloves, minced
- 4 medium tomatoes, seeded and chopped
- 1 jalapeno chili, seeded and chopped
- 1 cup fresh corn kernels
- 1 cup canned black beans, rinsed and drained
- ½ cup fresh cilantro, chopped
- 8 corn tortillas
- ½ cup smoke-flavored salsa

Preparation:
1. Add the olive oil to a saucepan, then heat it over medium heat.
2. Stir in the onion and sauté until soft.
3. Add the zucchini and the squash. Cook for 5 minutes.
4. Stir in the corn kernels, jalapeno, garlic, beans, and tomatoes.
5. Cook for another 5 minutes.
6. Stir in the cilantro, then remove the pan from the heat.
7. Warm each tortilla in a dry non-stick skillet for 20 seconds per side.
8. Place the tortillas on serving plates.
9. Spoon the vegetable mixture onto each tortilla.
10. Top the mixture with salsa.
11. Serve.
Serving Suggestion: Serve the meal with grilled avocados on the side.
Variation Tip: You can replace black beans with pinto beans.
Nutritional Information per Serving:
Calories 310 | Fat 6g |Sodium 97mg | Carbs 41g | Fiber 0.2g | Sugar 0.1g | Protein 10.5g

Beef Stroganoff

Prep Time: 10 minutes
Cook Time: 15 minutes
Serves: 2
Ingredients:
- ½ cup onion
- ½-pound boneless beef (fat removed)
- 4 cups yolkless egg noodles
- ½ can fat-free cream of mushroom
- 1 tablespoon all-purpose flour
- ½ teaspoon paprika
- ⅛ teaspoon black pepper
- ⅛ teaspoon white pepper
- ½ cup fat-free sour cream

Preparation:
1. Sauté the onions in a nonstick pan till the onions become translucent.
2. Add the beef into the pan and continue cooking till the beef turns brown and is tender.
3. Take the beef from the heat once cooked. Fill a large pot with water and bring the water to a boil. Place noodles into the pot and cook as per the packet directions.
4. Drain with cold water once the noodles are cooked. Add the soup mixture to the nonstick pan.
5. Add the salt, black pepper, white pepper and paprika to the soup mixture.
6. Add the beef into this mixture as well, and once the mixture is warmed, remove it from heat.
7. Add the sour cream after removing it from heat.
Serving Suggestion: Serve alongside green beans.
Variation Tip: Add in chili for a spicier result.
Nutritional Information per Serving:
Calories 391 | Fat 23g | Sodium 163mg | Carbs 21g | Fiber 1.3g | Sugar 2g | Protein 25g

Whole Grain Bruschetta

Prep Time: 10 minutes
Cook Time: 20 minutes
Serves: 2
Ingredients:
- 4 slices of wholegrain baguette (approx. 2 cm thick)
- 2 medium-sized tasty tomatoes

- 5 small Mozzarella balls
- 1 teaspoon parsley (chopped)
- 6 basil leaves
- 1 clove of garlic (chopped)
- ½ fennel (cut into cubes)
- 1 tablespoon olive oil
- 1 dash of Balsamic vinegar
- 1 pinch of black pepper

Preparation:
1. Rinse tomatoes and cut them into small cubes. If you prefer a dry topping, remove the seeds from the tomatoes beforehand.
2. Wash the fennel and cut it into small cubes. Chop the herbs and the clove of garlic.
3. Put all ingredients in a bowl, season with olive oil, Balsamic vinegar, and pepper. Stir well.
4. Cut the whole grain baguette in approx. Cut 2 cm slices and toast.
5. Halve the mozzarella balls and arrange them on the toast with the tomatoes.

Serving Suggestion: Garnish with arugula.
Variation Tip: Alternatively use wild garlic leaves in place of the garlic cloves.
Nutritional Information per Serving:
Calories 206 | Fat 4g | Sodium 109mg | Carbs 35g | Fiber 2g | Sugar 0.2g | Protein 7g

Baked Chicken and Wild Rice

Prep Time: 10 minutes + soaking time
Cook Time: 1 hour
Serves: 3
Ingredients:
- ½ pound boneless, skinless chicken breast halves, cut into 1-inch pieces
- ¾ cup whole pearl onions
- 1 cup unsalted chicken broth
- ¾ cup chopped celery
- ½ teaspoon chopped fresh tarragon
- 12 tablespoons uncooked wild rice
- ¾ cup dry white wine

Preparation:
1. Place chicken, onions, celery, ½ cup broth, and tarragon in a pan.
2. Place the pan over medium flame and cook until chicken is tender. Turn off the heat.
3. Combine white rice, wild rice, ½ cup broth, and dry white wine in a baking dish. Cover and set aside for 30 minutes to soak.
4. Stir chicken and vegetable mixture into the baking dish of rice mixture. Cover the dish with foil and place it in an oven that has been preheated to 300° F and bake until rice is tender.
5. It should take 45 – 50 minutes. I
6. if there is no broth in the baking dish and the rice is not cooked, add more broth.

7. Divide into three plates and serve.
Serving Suggestion: Garnish with chopped parsley.
Variation Tip: Substitute chicken broth with vegetable broth.
Nutritional Information per Serving:
Calories 313 | Fat 3g | Sodium 104mg | Carbs 38g | Fiber 3g | Sugar 5g | Protein 23g

Veggie Curry

Prep Time: 6 minutes
Cook Time: 10 minutes
Serves: 3
Ingredients:
- ½ medium onion
- 1½ garlic cloves, chopped finely
- 1½ medium carrots, peeled and sliced thinly
- 2 tablespoons water
- 1½ tablespoon fresh basil leaves, chopped
- 1 tablespoon olive oil
- ½ tablespoon fresh ginger, chopped finely
- 1¼ teaspoon curry powder
- ½ cup low-fat sour cream
- 1 medium bell pepper, seeded and sliced
- Fresh ground black pepper to taste

Preparation:
1. Take a large pan, heat the oil over medium-high heat and fry the onion for about four to five minutes.
2. Add ginger, garlic and curry powder and fry them for about a minute.
3. Add bell peppers and carrots and fry them for about three to four minutes.
4. Then, add sour cream and water and stir them well to combine.
5. Cook for about three to four minutes and stir occasionally.
6. Stir in black pepper and remove from heat.
7. Serve hot and enjoy!

Serving Suggestions: Garnish basil before serving.
Variation Tip: Add some vegetables like beans or cabbage.
Nutritional Information per Serving:
Calories: 163 | Fat: 13g | Sat Fat: 5.7g | Carbohydrates: 11g | Fiber: 2.1g | Sugar: 4.4g | Protein: 2.4g

Tomato and Green Bean Soup

Prep Time: 10 minutes
Cook Time: 35 minutes
Servings: 9
Ingredients:
- 1 cup onion, chopped
- 1 cup carrots, chopped
- 2 teaspoons butter
- 6 cups reduced-sodium chicken or vegetable broth
- 1 pound fresh green beans, cut into 1-inch pieces
- 1 garlic clove, minced
- 3 cups fresh tomatoes, diced
- ¼ cup fresh basil, minced or 1 tablespoon dried basil
- ½ teaspoon salt
- ¼ teaspoon pepper

Preparation:
1. Sauté the onion and carrots in butter in a large pot for 5 minutes.
2. Add the broth, beans, and garlic and bring to a boil.
3. Reduce the heat to low, cover, and cook for 20 minutes, or until the vegetables are soft.
4. Add the tomatoes, basil, salt, and pepper to taste. Cover and continue to cook for another 5 minutes.
5. Serve and enjoy!

Serving Suggestion: Season with salt and pepper before serving.
Variation Tip: You can add vegetables of your choice.
Nutritional Information per Serving:
Calories: 58|Fat: 1g|Sat Fat: 1g|Carbohydrates: 10g|Fiber: 3g|Sugar: 5g|Protein: 4g

Pasta & Beans Stew

Prep Time: 8 minutes
Cook Time: 25 minutes
Serves: 2
Ingredients:
- ½ large onion, chopped
- ½ bell pepper, seeded and chopped
- 1 tablespoon mixed fresh herbs, chopped
- 1 cup low-sodium vegetable broth
- ½ cup whole-wheat Rotini pasta

- ½ cup fresh collard greens
- ½ medium zucchini, chopped
- ½ tablespoon canola oil
- ½ teaspoon garlic, chopped finely
- 1 cup tomato, chopped finely
- ½ teaspoon Cayenne pepper
- 1 cup cooked Cannellini beans
- 1 teaspoon apple cider vinegar
- Fresh ground black pepper to taste

Preparation:
1. Take a large pan, heat oil over medium heat and fry onion, zucchini, bell peppers for about four to five minutes.
2. Add garlic, bay leaves, herbs and Cayenne pepper and fry them for about one minute.
3. Add broth and tomato and bring it to a boil.
4. Reduce the heat to low and gently cook while covered for about 15-20 minutes.
5. Stir in pasta and simmer, covered for about ten to 12 minutes.
6. Uncover and stir in remaining ingredients and simmer for about three to four minutes.
7. Serve hot and enjoy!

Serving Suggestions: Serve with crusty bread.
Variation Tip: A mix of chopped onion, carrots and celery may be substitute for the onions.
Nutritional Information per Serving:
Calories: 454 | Fat: 5.2g | Sat Fat: 0.4g | Carbohydrates: 78.4g | Fiber: 27.7g | Sugar: 8.9g | Protein: 27g

Roasted Lemon Swordfish

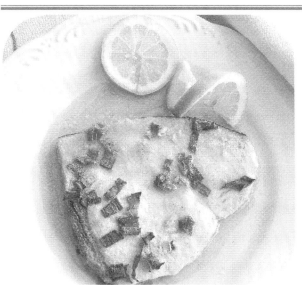

Prep Time: 10 minutes
Cook Time: 1 hour and 10 minutes
Serves: 4
Ingredients:
- 2 lemons, quartered, seeds removed
- 4 swordfish fillets, 6 ounces each
- ½ teaspoon canola oil
- ½ teaspoon garlic, chopped
- ¼ cup parsley, chopped

Preparation:
1. Preheat the oven to 375°F.
2. Toss the lemon wedges with the sugar in a bowl.
3. Spread this mixture in the baking dish and cover it with an aluminum sheet.
4. Roast the lemons for 1 hour until slightly brown.
5. Preheat the broiler and place its rack 4 inches below the heat source.

6. Place the fish in a baking tray and brush it with the canola oil.
7. Top the fish with the garlic and broil for 5 minutes per side.
8. Squeeze the juice from 1 roasted lemon on the fish.
9. Garnish with the parsley and remaining roasted lemon wedges.
Serving Suggestion: Serve the meal with roasted asparagus on the side.
Variation Tip: Add crushed red pepper on top before serving.
Nutritional Information per Serving:
Calories 280 | Fat 15g |Sodium 145mg | Carbs 9g | Fiber 1.4g | Sugar 3g | Protein 33g

Sardine with Olives

Prep Time: 6 minutes
Cook Time: 20 minutes
Serves: 2
Ingredients:
• 6 fresh sardines, cleaned and scaled
• 1 tablespoon olive oil
• 1 cup fresh parsley leaves, chopped
• 1 tablespoon capers, drained
• ½ tablespoon fresh oregano, chopped
• ¼ cup green olives, pitted and chopped
• ½ teaspoon fresh lemon zest, grated finely
• 1 garlic clove, thinly sliced
• Pinch of salt
• Fresh ground black pepper to taste
Preparation:
1. Preheat the oven to 400° F.
2. Season the sardines with salt and black pepper lightly.
3. In a large pan, heat the oil over medium heat and cook the sardines for about three minutes.
4. Flip the sardines and stir in the remaining ingredients.
5. Now, transfer it into oven and bake for about five minutes.
6. Remove from oven.
7. Serve hot and enjoy!
Serving Suggestions: Serve it lemons and hot sauce.
Variation Tip: Use ginger to combat the odor of fish.
Nutritional Information per Serving:
Calories: 229 | Fat: 15.8g | Sat Fat: 2.2g | Carbohydrates: 3.6g | Fiber: 1.7g | Sugar: 0.4g | Protein: 19g

Chicken & Veggie Parcel

Prep Time: 10 minutes
Cook Time: 30 minutes
Serves: 1
Ingredients:
• 1 cup tomato, seeded and chopped
• 1 cup zucchini, sliced thinly
• Fresh ground black pepper to taste
• 1 teaspoon garlic, minced
• 2 tablespoons fresh rosemary, minced
• 1½ teaspoon olive oil
• 4 ounces skinless, boneless chicken breast, chopped finely
• ½ cup fresh beans, trimmed and cut into 1-inch pieces
• Pinch of salt
Preparation:
1. Preheat the oven to 425° F.
2. Take a bowl and add all the ingredients and toss to coat well.
3. Place two large pieces of foil onto a smooth surface.
4. Place the chicken mixture in the center of each piece of foil evenly.
5. Loosely, wrap each foil around chicken mixture and secure tightly to form a parcel.
6. Place parcels in a baking-dish and bake them for about 25-30 minutes.
7. Remove the baking-dish from the oven and place parcels onto a platter.
8. Carefully open each parcel and serve.
Serving Suggestions: Serve it with rice and garnish coriander.
Variation Tip: You can also serve chicken parcels with a cold tomato sauce.
Nutritional Information per Serving:
Calories: 296 | Fat: 12.7g | Sat Fat: 3.1g | Carbohydrates: 19.9g | Fiber: 8.2g | Sugar: 7.5g | Protein: 29.8g

Beef and Blue Cheese Penne

Prep Time: 10 minutes
Cook Time: 20 minutes
Servings: 4
Ingredients:
- 2 cups uncooked whole-wheat penne pasta
- 2 beef tenderloin steaks
- ¼ teaspoon salt
- ¼ teaspoon pepper
- 5 ounces fresh baby spinach, coarsely chopped
- 2 cups grape tomatoes, halved
- ⅓ cup prepared pesto
- ¼ cup walnuts, chopped
- ¼ cup gorgonzola cheese, crumbled

Preparation:
1. Cook the pasta according to the packet instructions.
2. Season the steaks with salt and pepper. Grill the steaks in a grill pan over medium heat for 5–7 minutes on each side or until desired doneness is reached, or broil them 4 inches from the flame.
3. Drain the pasta and place it in a large mixing bowl. Toss in the spinach, tomatoes, pesto, and walnuts to coat.
4. Thinly slice the steak. Serve the pasta mixture with the steak and the cheese on top.
5. Serve and enjoy!

Serving Suggestion: Sprinkle with fresh chopped cilantro.
Variation Tip: You can use cherry tomatoes.
Nutritional Information per Serving:
Calories: 532|Fat: 22g|Sat Fat: 6g|Carbohydrates: 48g|Fiber: 9g|Sugar: 3g|Protein: 35g

Tilapia With Pineapple Salsa

Prep Time: 10 minutes
Cook Time: 20 minutes
Servings: 8
Ingredients:
- 2 cups pineapple, cubed
- 2 green onions, chopped
- ¼ cup green pepper, chopped
- ¼ cup cilantro, minced
- 6 tablespoons lime juice, divided
- ⅛ teaspoon plus ¼ teaspoon salt, divided
- Dash of cayenne pepper
- 1 tablespoon canola oil
- 8 tilapia fillets
- ⅛ teaspoon pepper

Preparation:
1. Combine the pineapple, green onions, green pepper, cilantro, 4 tablespoons of lime juice, ⅛ teaspoon of salt, and cayenne in a small bowl for the salsa. Refrigerate until ready to serve.
2. Drizzle the remaining lime juice and oil over the fillets, then season with the remaining salt and pepper.
3. Cover and grill the fish on an oiled rack over medium heat or broil them 4 inches from the flame until the fish just begins to flake easily with a fork, 2–3 minutes per side. Serve with a side of your prepared salsa.
4. Serve and enjoy!

Serving Suggestion: Serve with lemon wedges.
Variation Tip: You can use olive oil.
Nutritional Information per Serving:
Calories: 131|Fat: 3g|Sat Fat: 1g|Carbohydrates: 6g|Fiber: 1g|Sugar: 3g|Protein: 21g

Tuna Kabobs

Prep Time: 10 minutes
Cook Time: 25 minutes
Servings: 4
Ingredients:
- 1 pound tuna steaks, cut into 1-inch cubes
- 1 teaspoon coarsely ground pepper
- 2 large sweet red peppers, cut into 2x1-inch pieces
- 1 medium mango, cut into cubes

Preparation:
1. Season the tuna with salt and pepper. Thread the red peppers, tuna, and mango alternately on four metal or moistened wooden skewers.
2. The skewers should be placed on a greased grill pan. Cook, covered, over medium heat for 10-12 minutes, or until the tuna is slightly pink in the center and the peppers are cooked.
3. Serve and enjoy!

Serving Suggestion: Serve with salsa.
Variation Tip: You can add onions too.
Nutritional Information per Serving:
Calories: 205|Fat: 2g|Sat Fat: 0g|Carbohydrates: 20g|Fiber: 14|Sugar: 6g|Protein: 29g

Black Bean Frittata

Prep Time: 20 minutes
Cook Time: 15 minutes
Servings: 6
Ingredients:
- 6 large eggs
- 3 large egg whites
- ¼ cup salsa
- 1 tablespoon fresh parsley, minced
- ¼ teaspoon salt
- ¼ teaspoon pepper
- 1 tablespoon olive oil
- $1/3$ cup green pepper, chopped
- $1/3$ cup sweet red pepper, chopped
- 3 green onions, finely chopped
- 2 garlic cloves, minced
- 1 cup canned black beans, rinsed
- ½ cup white cheddar cheese, shredded

Preparation:
1. Preheat the oven to broil. Mix the first six ingredients in a bowl until well combined.
2. Heat the oil in a 10-inch ovenproof skillet over medium-high heat. Add the peppers and green onions and cook, occasionally stirring, for 3–4 minutes, or until the peppers are soft.
3. Cook for a further minute after adding the garlic. Add the beans and mix well.
4. Reduce the heat to medium-low and whisk in the egg mixture. Cook for 4–6 minutes, uncovered, or until the eggs are nearly set. Sprinkle with the cheese.
5. Broil 3–4 inches from the heat source for 3–4 minutes or until the frittata is light golden brown and the eggs are completely set. Let the frittata stand for 5 minutes.
6. Serve and enjoy!

Serving Suggestion: Serve with salsa.
Variation Tip: You can top with sliced olives.
Nutritional Information per Serving:
Calories: 183|Fat: 10g|Sat Fat: 4g|Carbohydrates: 9g|Fiber: 2g|Sugar: 2g|Protein: 13g

Turkey and Vegetable Barley Soup

Prep Time: 10 minutes
Cook Time: 25 minutes
Servings: 6
Ingredients:
- 1 tablespoon canola oil
- 5 medium carrots, chopped
- 1 medium onion, chopped
- $2/3$ cup quick-cooking barley
- 6 cups reduced-sodium chicken broth
- 2 cups cooked turkey breast, cubed
- 2 cups fresh baby spinach
- ½ teaspoon pepper

Preparation:
1. Heat the oil in a saucepan over medium heat. Add the carrots and cook until they're crisp-tender, about 4–5 minutes.
2. Add the barley and broth and bring the mixture to a boil. Reduce the heat to low, then cover and cook for 10–15 minutes, or until the carrots and barley are softened. Add the turkey, spinach, and pepper and cook until they're heated through.
3. Serve and enjoy!

Serving Suggestion: Add some fresh herbs on top.
Variation Tip: You can also add mushrooms.
Nutritional Information per Serving:
Calories: 208|Fat: 4g|Sat Fat: 1g|Carbohydrates: 23g|Fiber: 6g|Sugar: 4g|Protein: 21g

Skillet Cabbage Roll

Prep Time: 10 minutes
Cook Time: 20 minutes
Servings: 6
Ingredients:
- 1 can (28 ounces) whole plum tomatoes, undrained
- 1 pound extra-lean ground beef
- 1 large onion, chopped
- 1 can (8 ounces) tomato sauce
- 2 tablespoons cider vinegar

- 1 tablespoon brown sugar
- 1 teaspoon dried oregano
- 1 teaspoon dried thyme
- ½ teaspoon pepper
- 1 small head cabbage, thinly sliced
- 1 medium green bell pepper

Preparation:

1. Drain the tomatoes, set aside the juice, then finely slice the tomatoes.
2. Cook the beef and onion in a large non-stick skillet over medium-high heat for 6–8 minutes, or until the meat is no longer pink, breaking up beef into crumbles.
3. Combine the tomato sauce, vinegar, brown sugar, seasonings, chopped tomatoes, and the conserved tomato liquid in a mixing bowl.
4. Add the tomato mixture to the skillet and cook for 6 minutes, covered, with the cabbage and pepper, stirring periodically.
5. Cook for an additional 6–8 minutes, uncovered, or until the cabbage is tender.
6. Serve and enjoy!

Serving Suggestion: Serve with brown rice.
Variation Tip: You can also add red bell pepper.
Nutritional Information per Serving:
Calories: 332|Fat: 5g|Sat Fat: 2g|Carbohydrates: 50g|Fiber: 9g|Sugar: 12g|Protein: 22g

Basil Turkey Burgers

Prep Time: 10 minutes
Cook Time: 25 minutes
Servings: 6
Ingredients:
- ¼ cup chopped fresh basil
- 3 tablespoons mesquite smoke-flavored barbecue sauce
- 2 tablespoons quick-cooking oats or oat bran
- 1 garlic clove, minced
- ¼ teaspoon garlic salt
- ⅛ teaspoon pepper
- 1 pound lean ground turkey
- 4 whole-wheat or multigrain hamburger buns, split

Preparation:

1. Combine the basil, barbecue sauce, oats, garlic, garlic salt, and pepper in a large mixing bowl. Add the turkey and stir briefly but thoroughly. Form four 1/2-inch-thick patties from the mixture.

2. Grill the burgers, covered, over medium heat for 5–7 minutes on each side on a lightly greased grill pan.
3. Grill the buns cut side down for 30–60 seconds over medium heat. Serve the burgers on the buns with your favorite toppings.
4. Serve and enjoy!

Serving Suggestion: Serve with sweet potato fries.
Variation Tip: You can also add fresh basil leaves.
Nutritional Information per Serving:
Calories: 315|Fat: 11g|Sat Fat: 3g|Carbohydrates: 29g|Fiber: 4g|Sugar: 8g|Protein: 27g

Black Bean and Sweet Potato Rice Bowls

Prep Time: 10 minutes
Cook Time: 25 minutes
Servings: 6
Ingredients:
- ¾ cup uncooked long-grain rice
- ¼ teaspoon garlic salt
- 1½ cups water
- 3 tablespoons olive oil, divided
- 1 large sweet potato, peeled and diced
- 1 medium red onion, finely chopped
- 4 cups fresh kale, chopped
- 1 can black beans, rinsed and drained
- 2 tablespoons sweet chili sauce

Preparation:

1. In a large saucepan, combine the rice, garlic salt, and water; bring to a boil. Reduce the heat to low; cover and cook for 15–20 minutes, or until the water is absorbed and the rice is soft. Remove from the heat and set aside for 5 minutes.
2. Meanwhile, heat 2 tablespoons of oil in a large skillet over medium-high heat and sauté the sweet potato for 8 minutes.
3. Cook and stir until the potato is cooked, about 4–6 minutes.
4. Add the kale and cook, frequently stirring, until the kale is soft, about 3–5 minutes. Add the beans and heat thoroughly.
5. Add 2 tablespoons of chili sauce and the remaining oil to the rice, gently stirring, then add to the potato mixture.
6. Serve and enjoy!

Serving Suggestion: Serve with lime wedges.
Variation Tip: You can also add additional sweet chili sauce.
Nutritional Information per Serving:
Calories: 435|Fat: 11g|Sat Fat: 2g|Carbohydrates: 74g|Fiber: 8g|Sugar: 10g|Protein: 10g

Chickpea Mint Tabbouleh

Prep Time: 10 minutes
Cook Time: 25 minutes
Servings: 4
Ingredients:
• 1 cup bulgur
• 2 cups water
• 1 cup fresh or frozen peas, thawed
• 1 can chickpeas, rinsed and drained
• ½ cup fresh parsley, minced
• ¼ cup fresh mint, minced
• ¼ cup olive oil
• 2 tablespoons soft sun-dried tomatoes (not packed in oil), julienned
• 2 tablespoons lemon juice
• ½ teaspoon salt
• ¼ teaspoon pepper
Preparation:
1. Combine the bulgur and water in a large saucepan and bring to a boil. Reduce the heat to low and cook for 10 minutes, covered.
2. Stir in the fresh or thawed peas and cook, covered, for 5 minutes, or until the bulgur and peas are soft.
3. Place in a large mixing bowl. Add and combine the remaining ingredients.
4. Serve warm and enjoy!
Serving Suggestion: Sprinkle fresh cilantro on top.
Variation Tip: You can refrigerate the dish and serve it cold.
Nutritional Information per Serving:
Calories: 380|Fat: 15g|Sat Fat: 2g|Carbohydrates: 51g|Fiber: 11g|Sugar: 6g|Protein: 11g

Ricotta, Tomato, and Corn Pasta

Prep Time: 10 minutes
Cook Time: 25 minutes
Servings: 8
Ingredients:
• 3 cups uncooked whole-wheat elbow macaroni (about 12 ounces)
• 1 can (15 ounces) cannellini beans, rinsed and drained
• 2 cups cherry tomatoes, halved
• 1 cup fresh or frozen corn, thawed
• ½ cup red onion, finely chopped
• ½ cup part-skim ricotta cheese
• ¼ cup parmesan cheese, grated
• 2 tablespoons fresh basil, minced
• 1 tablespoon olive oil
• 3 garlic cloves, minced
• 1 teaspoon salt
• 1 teaspoon fresh rosemary, chopped
• ½ teaspoon pepper
• 3 cups arugula or baby spinach
Preparation:
1. Cook the pasta according to the packet directions. Drain carefully after rinsing with cold water.
2. Combine the beans, tomatoes, corn, onion, ricotta, parmesan, basil, oil, garlic, salt, rosemary, and pepper in a large mixing bowl.
3. Add the pasta and mix well. Toss in the arugula lightly to combine.
4. Serve and enjoy!
Serving Suggestion: Sprinkle chopped fresh parsley on top.
Variation Tip: You can use dried rosemary instead of minced fresh rosemary.
Nutritional Information per Serving:
Calories: 275| **at:** 5g|Sat Fat: 1g|Carbohydrates: 46g|Fiber: 8g|Sugar: 44|Protein: 13g

Pork Chops with Tomato Curry

Prep Time: 15 minutes
Cook Time: 25 minutes
Servings: 6
Ingredients:
• 4 teaspoons butter, divided
• 6 boneless pork loin chops
• 1 small onion, finely chopped
• 3 medium apples, thinly sliced
• 1 can (28 ounces) whole tomatoes, undrained
• 2 teaspoons stevia
• 2 teaspoons curry powder
• ½ teaspoon salt
• ½ teaspoon chili powder
• 4 cups brown rice, cooked (hot)
Preparation:

1. Melt 2 teaspoons of butter in a stockpot over medium-high heat. Add the pork chops in batches and brown them. Remove from the pan.
2. Heat the remaining butter in the same pan over medium heat. Add the onion and cook, stirring, for 2–3 minutes, or until the onion is soft.
3. Combine the apples, tomatoes, stevia, curry powder, salt, and chili powder in a large mixing bowl.
4. Add the mixture to the pan and bring it to a boil, stirring to break up the tomatoes.
5. Return the pork chops to the pan. Reduce the heat to low and cook for 10 minutes, uncovered. Allow for 5 minutes of resting before serving.
6. Serve and enjoy!
Serving Suggestion: Serve with rice.
Variation Tip: You can also add toasted slivered almonds.
Nutritional Information per Serving:
Calories: 478|Fat: 14g|Sat Fat: 5g|Carbohydrates: 50g|Fiber: 7g|Sugar: 15g|Protein: 38g

Spiced Salmon

Prep Time: 10 minutes
Cook Time: 20 minutes
Servings: 8
Ingredients:
- 1 tablespoon stevia
- 1 tablespoon soy sauce
- 1 tablespoon butter, melted
- 1 tablespoon olive oil
- ½ teaspoon garlic powder
- ½ ground mustard
- ½ teaspoon paprika
- ½ teaspoon pepper
- ¼ teaspoon dill weed
- Dash of salt
- Dash of dried tarragon
- Dash of cayenne pepper
- 1 salmon fillet (2 pounds)
Preparation:
1. Combine all the ingredients except the salmon in a bowl.
2. Brush the salmon with the mixture.
3. Place the salmon, skin side down, on a lightly greased grill rack or baking sheet.
4. Broil the salmon 4 inches below the heat source for 10–15 minutes, or until the salmon just begins to flake easily with a fork.
5. Serve and enjoy!
Serving Suggestion: Sprinkle with chopped fresh cilantro.
Variation Tip: You can skip the stevia.

Nutritional Information per Serving:
Calories: 256|Fat: 17g|Sat Fat: 4g|Carbohydrates: 5g|Fiber: 0g|Sugar: 4g|Protein: 20g

Shrimp Orzo With Feta

Prep Time: 10 minutes
Cook Time: 20 minutes
Servings: 4
Ingredients:
- 1¼ cups uncooked whole-wheat orzo pasta
- 2 tablespoons olive oil
- 2 garlic cloves, minced
- 2 medium tomatoes, chopped
- 2 tablespoons lemon juice
- 1¼ pounds uncooked shrimp, peeled and deveined
- 2 tablespoons fresh cilantro, minced
- ¼ teaspoon pepper
- ½ cup feta cheese, crumbled
Preparation:
1. Cook the orzo as directed on the packet.
2. Meanwhile, heat the oil in a skillet. Add the garlic and cook for 1 minute, stirring constantly. Toss in the tomatoes and the lemon juice and bring the mixture to a boil.
3. Add the shrimp and mix well. Reduce the heat to low and cook, uncovered, for 4–5 minutes, or until the shrimp turn pink.
4. Drain the orzo. Heat through the orzo, cilantro, and pepper in the shrimp mixture.
5. Serve and enjoy!
Serving Suggestion: Sprinkle with the crumbled feta cheese.
Variation Tip: You can also add chopped onions.
Nutritional Information per Serving:
Calories: 406|Fat: 12g|Sat Fat: 3g|Carbohydrates: 40g|Fiber: 9g|Sugar: 2g|Protein: 33g

Veggie Chili

Prep Time: 10 minutes
Cook Time: 1 hour 30 minutes
Serves: 4
Ingredients:
- ½ yellow onion, chopped
- ¼ cup carrot, peeled and chopped
- 1 garlic clove, minced
- 1 tablespoon red chili powder
- ¼ cup green bell pepper, seeded and chopped
- ½ can salt-free tomato paste
- ½ tablespoon ground cumin
- 2 ounces fresh mushrooms, sliced
- Pinch of salt
- Fresh ground black pepper to taste

Preparation:
1. Take a large pan and heat over medium-high and cook for about eight to ten minutes.
2. Drain the excess grease from the pan.
3. Stir in remaining ingredients and bring to a boil.
4. Reduce the heat to low and cook while covered for about three hours.
5. Serve hot and enjoy!

Serving Suggestions: Serve it with cornbread croutons as a topping.
Variation Tip: You can store it in a plastic bag or can and use it later on.
Nutritional Information per Serving:
Calories: 252 | Fat: 7.7g | Sat Fat: 2.8g | Carbohydrates: 8.6g | Fiber: 2.3g | Sugar: 4.3g | Protein: 36.5g

Chicken with Broccoli & Mushrooms

Prep Time: 10 minutes
Cook Time: 25 minutes
Serves: 3
Ingredients:
- ½ pound skinless, boneless chicken breast, cubed
- 2 tablespoons water
- 3 garlic cloves, minced
- 1½ tablespoon olive oil
- ½ medium onion, chopped
- 8 ounces small broccoli florets
- Pinch of salt
- Fresh ground black pepper to taste

Preparation:
1. Heat the oil in a large frying-pan over medium heat and cook the chicken cubes for about four to five minutes.
2. With a spoon, transfer the chicken cubes onto a plate.
3. In the same frying pan, add the onion and fry for about four to five minutes.
4. Add the mushrooms and cook for about four to five minutes.
5. Stir in the cooked chicken, broccoli and water and cook it while covered for about eight to ten minutes, stirring occasionally.
6. Stir in salt and black pepper and remove from heat.
7. Serve hot.

Serving Suggestions: Serve it with white rice.
Variation Tip: You can also use thinly sliced steak instead of chicken.
Nutritional Information per Serving:
Calories: 1646 | Fat: 89.7g | Sat Fat: 2g | Carbohydrates: 64.1g | Fiber: 24.5g | Sugar: 0.8g | Protein: 147.9g

Grilled Asparagus

Prep Time: 10 minutes
Cook Time: 3 minutes
Serves: 4
Ingredients:
- 5 tablespoons extra virgin olive oil
- 1 pound asparagus, ends trimmed
- Grated zest of 1 large lemon
- Juice of ½ lemon
- 3 large cloves garlic, minced
- ¼ teaspoon Sea salt
- ⅛ teaspoon cracked black pepper

Preparation:
1. In a large baking dish or rimmed cookie sheets, lay the spears in a single, even layer and drizzle with oil.
2. Roll the spears in the oil to coat evenly.
3. Add the lemon zest, lemon juice, garlic, salt, and pepper over the top. Roll the spears again to coat all sides with the seasonings.
4. Place on a hot grill, and rotate the spears constantly, so they do not burn.
5. Grill for about 2 minutes or to desired tenderness, and then return to marinating pan to serve.

Serving Suggestion: Serve with lemon slices.
Variation Tip: Substitute the lemon zest and juice with lime.
Nutritional Information per Serving:
Calories 163 | Fat 18 g | Sodium 292 mg | Carbs 3 g | Fiber0.9 g | Sugar 0 g | Protein 1 g

Kale Chips with Feta

Prep Time: 10 minutes
Cook Time: 25 minutes
Serves: 4
Ingredients:
- 1 large bunch curly green kale, stems and midrib removed
- 1 tablespoon grapeseed oil
- 2 tablespoons grated Feta
- Dash of salt
- 1 teaspoon curry powder

Preparation:
1. Preheat the oven to 300° F.
2. Line 2 large baking sheets with aluminum foil.
3. Discard the stem and pull out the tough midrib from the kale leaves. Roughly tear the leaves into large pieces.
4. Wash the leaves and pat dry with a paper towel. Place the leaves in a large bowl and spritz with the oil.
5. Use your hands to massage the oil into the leaves.
6. Sprinkle with the Feta, salt, and curry powder and toss to combine well, working it into the kale to ensure it is coated completely.
7. Spread the kale out evenly into a single layer on the baking sheets, being certain not to overcrowd the kale.
8. Place the kale in the oven and bake for 10 minutes, then flip the baking sheet and continue baking for a further 10 to 15 minutes. The kale will shrink as it firms up and get crispy, and the edges will begin to brown slightly.
9. Off heat, remove the kale from the oven, and let the stand cool slightly, 3 to 5 minutes, before enjoying.

Serving Suggestion: Top with pine nuts.
Variation Tip: The key to perfect kale chips is baking them at a lower temperature; increasing the temperature will burn.
Nutritional Information per Serving:
Calories 79 | Fat 5 g | Sodium 92 mg | Carbs 7 g | Fiber 3 g | Sugar 2 g | Protein 3 g

Roasted Carrots and Beets

Prep Time: 10 minutes
Cook Time: 1 hour
Serves: 4
Ingredients:
- Nonstick cooking spray
- 8 medium carrots, peeled
- 4 medium beets, peeled
- 4 tablespoons extra-virgin olive oil, divided
- 2 tablespoons Balsamic vinegar, divided
- 2 tablespoons chopped fresh parsley, divided
- 1 teaspoon grated lemon zest
- ⅛ teaspoon freshly ground black pepper

Preparation:
1. Preheat the oven to 375° F.

111

2. Line a sheet pan with aluminum foil and coat with nonstick cooking spray.
3. Cut the carrots diagonally into 2-inch lengths on the thin end of the carrot and 1-inch lengths on the thick end.
4. Cut the beets into 1- to 2-inch cubes. In a large bowl, whisk together two tablespoons of oil, one tablespoon of vinegar, and one tablespoon of parsley.
5. Add the carrots and toss. Place the carrots on half of the prepared sheet pan. Add the remaining two tablespoons of oil, one tablespoon of vinegar, and one tablespoon of parsley to the bowl.
6. Add the beets and toss. Place the beets on the other half of the prepared sheet pan.
7. Sprinkle with lemon zest and pepper.
8. Bake for about 1 hour, or until the beets turn a dark purple and the carrots a dull orange.
9. They should be soft enough to cut through with a fork.
Serving Suggestion: Garnish with rosemary sprigs.
Variation Tip: Other vegetables that will caramelize nicely are sweet potatoes, squash, and parsnips.
Nutritional Information per Serving:
Calories 238 | Fat 18g | Sodium 151mg | Carbs 21g | Fiber 6g | Sugar 4g | Protein 2g

Baked Cheese Envelopes

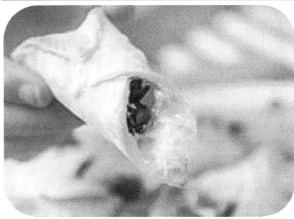

Prep Time: 30 minutes
Cook Time: 15 minutes
Serves: 12
Ingredients
• ½ cup fresh or frozen cranberries
• ½ medium orange, quartered
• 2 tbsp. sugar
• 1 cinnamon stick
• 1 sheet puff pastry dough, cut into 12¼-oz. squares
• 6 oz. soft mozzarella cheese, cut into ½-oz. cubes
• 2 tbsp. water
• 1 egg white
Preparation
1. Heat the oven to 425 F.
2. Heat a small sauté pan to medium-high heat and lightly coat it with cooking spray. Reduce the heat to low. Place the cranberries, orange, sugar, and cinnamon stick in the pan and cook for about 10 minutes, stirring constantly, until the cranberries are soft and the mixture starts to thicken. Remove from the heat and allow to cool. Remove the cinnamon stick and orange quarters.
3. Roll out each square of puff pastry. Place one cube of cheese and 1 tsp. of the cooled cranberry mixture onto each puff pastry square.
4. In a small bowl, combine the water and egg white. Using a pastry brush, dab a small amount of the egg

mixture onto the inside of the puff pastry. Pull one corner of the pastry at a time around the cheese and cranberry mixture like an envelope.
5. Baste the top of the pastry with the egg mixture. Place the envelopes on a baking sheet and bake for 10 to 12 minutes or until golden brown.
Serving Suggestion: Serve with tea.
Variation Tip: Prepare this appetizer the day before guests arrive. Keep wrapped in the fridge until ready to bake.
Nutritional Information Per Serving:
Calories 116 | Protein 4g | Carbohydrate 9g | Dietary fiber 0g | Sugars 4g | Fat 7g | Sodium 133mg

Lemony Kale & Carrot

Prep Time: 20 minutes
Cook Time: 15 minutes
Serves: 2
Ingredients:
• ½ small onion, chopped
• ¼ pound carrot, peeled and shredded
• ½ tablespoon fresh lemon juice
• 1 tablespoon olive oil
• 1½ garlic cloves, minced
• ½ pound fresh kale, tough ribs removed and chopped
• Pinch of salt
• Fresh ground black pepper to taste
Preparation:
1. Take a large frying-pan and heat the oil over medium heat and fry the onion or about four to five minutes.
2. Stir-in garlic and fry for about a minute.
3. Add the kale and cook for about three to four minutes.
4. Stir in the carrot, lemon juice, salt and black pepper and cook for about four to five minutes.
5. Serve hot and enjoy!
Serving Suggestions: Serve with lemon juice.
Variation Tip: You can store leftovers in refrigerator for up to 3 days.
Nutritional Information per Serving:
Calories: 150 | Fat: 7.1g | Sat Fat: 1g | Carbohydrates: 19.9g | Fiber: 3.5g | Sugar: 3.6g | Protein: 4.2g

Basil Pesto Stuffed Mushrooms

Prep Time: 5 minutes
Cook Time: 15 minutes
Serves: 20
Ingredients
• 20 cremini mushrooms, washed and stems removed
Topping:
• 1½ cups panko breadcrumbs
• ¼ cup melted butter
• 3 tbsp. chopped fresh parsley
Basil-Pesto Filling:
• 2 cups fresh basil leaves
• ¼ cup fresh parmesan cheese
• 2 tbsp. pumpkin seeds
• 1 tbsp. olive oil
• 1 tbsp. fresh garlic
• 2 tsp. lemon juice
• ½ tsp. kosher salt
Preparation
1. Heat the oven to 350°F. Line the mushroom caps upside down on a baking sheet.
2. To prepare the topping: In a small bowl, combine the panko, butter, and parsley. Set aside.
3. To prepare the filling: Place the basil, cheese, pumpkin seeds, oil, garlic, lemon juice, and salt in a food processor. Process until evenly mixed.
4. Generously stuff the mushroom caps with the basil-pesto filling. Sprinkle each mushroom with about 1 tsp. of the panko topping. Gently pat down the topping.
5. Bake for 10 to 15 minutes or until golden brown.
Serving Suggestion: Refrigerate until ready to serve.
Variation Tip: Add more spices, if desired.
Nutritional Information Per Serving:
Calories 59 | Protein 2g | Carbohydrate 4g | Dietary fiber 0g | Sugars 0g | Fat 3g | Sodium 80mg

Cilantro Rice

Prep Time: 10 minutes
Cook Time: 45 minutes
Serves: 4
Ingredients:

• 1 tablespoon extra-virgin olive oil
• 1 cup brown rice
• Zest and juice of 1 large lime
• 1½ cups water
• 2 tablespoons chopped fresh cilantro
Preparation:
1. In a medium pot, heat the oil over medium heat until warm.
2. Add the rice and lime zest and cook, occasionally stirring or toasting for 3 to 5 minutes.
3. Add the water and bring to a boil. Cover, reduce the heat to low, and simmer for about 45 minutes, or until the rice has absorbed all the water.
4. Serve.
Serving Suggestion: Stir in lime juice and cilantro.
Variation Tip: When in a rush, you can use precooked boil-in-a-bag rice, which usually cooks in 10 minutes. Just add the lime zest to the water and cook according to the package directions.
Nutritional Information per Serving:
Calories 202 | Fat 5g | Sodium 3mg | Carbs 36g | Fiber 2g | Sugar 4g| Protein 3.5g

Garlicky Carrots

Prep Time: 6 minutes
Cook Time: 8 minutes
Serves: 1
Ingredients:
• 1 tablespoon olive oil
• 1 garlic clove, minced
• ¼ pound carrots, peeled and sliced
• ½ onion, sliced
• ½ piece fresh ginger, grated
• Pinch of salt
• Fresh ground black pepper to taste
Preparation:
1. Take a bowl and stir all the ingredients together.
2. Cover the bowl and set aside for about 30 minutes.
3. Heat a frying pan over medium heat and cook the carrot mixture for about seven to eight minutes, stirring occasionally.
Serving Suggestions: Garnish with fresh parsley.
Variation Tip: Use high heat when roasting carrots.
Nutritional Information per Serving:
Calories: 196 | Fat: 14.1g | Sat Fat: 2g | Carbohydrates: 18g | Fiber: 4.2g | Sugar: 8g | Protein: 1.8g

Brown-Rice Pilaf

Prep Time: 10 minutes
Cook Time: 10 minutes
Serves: 4
Ingredients:
- 1 cup low-sodium vegetable broth
- 1 tablespoon olive oil
- 1 clove garlic, minced
- 1 scallion, thinly sliced
- 1 tablespoon minced onion flakes
- 1 cup instant brown rice
- Salt and black pepper

Preparation:
1. Mix the vegetable broth, olive oil, garlic, scallion, and minced onion flakes in a saucepan and let it boil.
2. Add rice, return mixture to boil, then reduce heat and simmer for 10 minutes.
3. Remove from heat and let stand for 5 minutes.
4. Fluff with a fork and season with black pepper.

Serving Suggestion: Garnish with parsley.
Variation Tip: Substitute vegetable broth with low-sodium chicken or beef broth.
Nutritional Information per Serving:
Calories 100 | Fat 2 g | Sodium 35 mg | Carbs 19 g | Fiber 2 g | Sugar 1 g | Protein 2 g

Zucchini Sticks

Prep Time: 10 minutes
Cook Time: 20 minutes
Serves: 2
Ingredients:
- 3 medium zucchinis, sliced into sticks
- 1 cup whole-wheat breadcrumbs
- ½ cup Parmesan cheese, grated
- 1 egg
- ¼ teaspoon salt
- ¼ teaspoon black pepper
- Optional: Ranch dressing or low-sodium Marinara sauce for dipping

Preparation:
1. Preheat oven to 400° F.
2. Line a baking pan with parchment paper set aside.
3. Slice the zucchinis into sticks. In a bowl, beat the eggs, season with salt and black pepper.

4. In a different bowl, combine the breadcrumbs with the Parmesan cheese, season with salt and pepper
5. Soak each zucchini stick into the egg wash and roll it in the breadcrumb mixture.
6. Arrange on the baking sheet, then bake until crispy and golden brown.

Serving Suggestion: Serve with Ranch dressing or Marinara sauce.
Variation Tip: for a vegan option, use vegan Parmesan.
Nutritional Information per Serving:
Calories 128 | Fat 7g | Sodium 286mg | Carbs 10g | Fiber 1g | Sugar 1g | Protein 6g

Roasted Butternut Squash Fries

Prep Time: 10 minutes
Cook Time: 40 minutes
Serves: 6
Ingredients
- 1 medium butternut squash
- 1 tbsp. olive oil
- 1 tbsp. chopped fresh thyme
- 1 tbsp. chopped fresh rosemary
- ½ tsp. salt

Preparation
1. Heat the oven to 425°F. Lightly coat a baking sheet with non-stick cooking spray.
2. Peel the skin from the butternut squash and cut into even sticks, about ½-inch wide and 3 inches long.
3. Combine the squash, oil, thyme, rosemary, and salt in a medium bowl. Mix until the squash is evenly coated.
4. Spread the mixture onto the baking sheet and roast for 10 minutes.
5. Remove the baking sheet from the oven and shake to loosen the squash. Place back in the oven and continue to roast for another 5 to 10 minutes until golden brown.

Serving Suggestion: Serve warm.
Variation Tip: To ensure even cooking, cut the vegetables into uniform sizes. This recipe also works with sweet potatoes or acorn squash.
Nutritional Information Per Serving:
Calories 62 | Protein 1g | Carbohydrate 11g | Dietary fiber 3g | Sugars 2g | Fat 2g | Sodium 168mg

Roast Mushrooms

Prep Time: 10 minutes
Cook Time: 30 minutes
Serves: 4
Ingredients:
• 2 tablespoons olive oil
• 10 ounces Pink oyster mushrooms
• Black pepper to taste
• 1 teaspoon fresh basil, chopped
• 1 teaspoon fresh thyme, finely chopped
• 1 sprig rosemary
• 2 tablespoons garlic, finely sliced
Preparation:
1. Preheat the oven to 400° F. Oil a baking tray, add all the ingredients except the garlic to the tray.
2. Toss well to coat the mushrooms fully.
3. Roast in the oven for about 25 minutes.
4. Remove from the oven, layer the garlic beneath the mushrooms, and roast for 5 minutes.
5. Serve hot and enjoy.
Serving Suggestion: Garnish with sprigs of rosemary.
Variation Tip: Feel free to use mushrooms of your choice.
Nutritional Information per Serving:
Calories 94 | Fat 7g | Sodium 253mg | Carbs 5g | Fiber 2g | Sugar 3g | Protein 5g

Sour Cream Green Beans

Prep Time: 10 minutes
Cook Time: 4 hours
Serves: 8
Ingredients:
• 15 ounces green beans
• 14 ounces corn
• 4 ounces mushrooms, sliced
• 11 ounces cream of mushroom soup, low-fat and sodium-free
• ½ cup low-fat sour cream
• ½ cup almonds, chopped
• ½ cup low-fat Cheddar cheese, shredded
Preparation:

1. In your slow cooker, mix the green beans with the corn, mushrooms soup, mushrooms, almonds, cheese and sour cream, toss
2. cover and cook on low for 4 hours.
3. Stir one more time, divide between plates and serve as a side dish.
Serving Suggestion: Top with a sprinkle of paprika.
Variation Tip: Substitute almonds with walnuts.
Nutritional Information per Serving:
Calories 360 | Fat 12.7g | Sodium 220mg | Carbs 58.3g | Fiber 10g | Sugar 10.3g | Protein 14g

Gingered Asparagus

Prep Time: 5 minutes
Cook Time: 6 minutes
Serves: 1
Ingredients:
• ½ tablespoon fresh ginger, minced
• ½ teaspoon cumin seeds
• 1 teaspoon fresh lemon juice
• 2 tablespoons olive oil
• ½ asparagus, trimmed and cut into 2-inch pieces
• Pinch of salt
• Fresh ground black pepper to taste
Preparation:
1. Take a frying-pan and heat oil over medium heat and fry cumin seeds for about a minute.
2. Add remaining ingredients and stir fry for about four to five minutes.
3. Serve warm and enjoy!
Serving Suggestions: Serve it with sesame seeds as topping.
Variation Tip: Use warm asparagus for a great taste.
Nutritional Information per Serving:
Calories: 268 | Fat: 28.5g | Sat Fat: 4.1g | Carbohydrates: 5.1g | Fiber: 1.9g | Sugar: 1.5g | Protein: 2g

Chickpeas Hummus

Prep Time: 10 minutes
Cook Time: 0 minutes
Serves: 7
Ingredients:
• 1 (15 ounces) can chickpeas, drained and rinsed

- 3 tablespoons sesame tahini
- 2 tablespoons olive oil
- 3 garlic cloves, chopped
- 1 lemon juice
- Salt and black pepper, to taste

Preparation:
1. In a food processor or blender, combine all the ingredients: until smooth but thick.
2. Add water, if necessary, to produce smoother hummus.
3. Store covered for up 5 days.

Serving Suggestion: Top with some chickpeas and chopped parsley.

Variation Tip: For red pepper hummus, simply add 1 chopped red pepper to the ingredients. Try beets, cucumber, olives, or avocado. The possibilities are endless.

Nutritional Information per Serving:
Calories 147 | Fat 10 g | Sodium 64 mg | Carbs 11 g | Fiber 4 g | Sugar 0 g | Protein 6 g

Fruit Salsa and Sweet Chips

Prep Time: 20 minutes
Cook Time: 10 minutes
Serves: 8
Ingredients
Tortilla Crisps:
- 8 whole-wheat, fat-free tortillas
- Cooking spray
- 1 tbsp. sugar
- ½ tbsp. cinnamon

Fruit Salsa:
- 3 cups diced fresh fruit, such as apples, oranges, kiwi, strawberries, grapes, or other fresh fruit
- 2 tbsp. sugar-free jelly, any flavor
- 1 tbsp. honey or agave nectar
- 2 tbsp. orange juice

Preparation
1. Heat the oven to 350°F. Cut each tortilla into 8 wedges. Lay the pieces on two baking sheets (make sure they aren't overlapping). Spray the tortilla pieces with cooking spray.
2. In a small bowl, combine the sugar and cinnamon. Sprinkle the mixture evenly over the tortilla wedges.
3. Bake for 10 to 12 minutes or until the pieces are crisp. Place on a cooling rack and let cool.
4. Cut the fruit into cubes. Gently mix the fruit together in a mixing bowl.
5. In another bowl, whisk together the jelly, honey, and orange juice. Pour this over the diced fruit. Mix gently.
6. Cover the bowl with plastic wrap and refrigerate for 2 to 3 hours.

Serving Suggestion: Serve the fruit as a dip or topping for the cinnamon tortilla chips.

Variation Tip: Sprinkle some toasted nuts over the top of the fruit.
Nutritional Information Per Serving:
Calories 105 | Protein 2g | Carbohydrate 24g | Dietary fiber 10g | Sugars 4g | Fat 0.1g | Sodium 181mg

Garlicky Broccoli

Prep Time: 5 minutes
Cook Time: 8 minutes
Serves: 1
Ingredients:
- ½ tablespoon olive oil
- 1 cup broccoli florets
- 1 tablespoon water
- 1 garlic clove, minced
- Fresh ground black pepper to taste
- Pinch of salt

Preparation:
1. Take a large frying pan, heat the oil over medium heat and fry the garlic for about a minute.
2. Add the broccoli and stir fry for two minutes.
3. Stir in water, salt and black pepper and stir fry for four to five minutes.
4. Carefully open each parcel and serve hot.

Serving Suggestions: Serve it with a light drizzle of fresh lemon juice.
Variation Tip: Cut the broccoli florets into small pieces.
Nutritional Information per Serving:
Calories: 96 | Fat: 7.3g | Sat Fat: 1g | Carbohydrates: 7.1g | Fiber: 2.5g | Sugar: 1.6g | Protein: 2.8g

Broccoli Black Bean Rice

Prep Time: 10 minutes
Cook Time: 30 minutes
Serves: 4
Ingredients:
- 1 cup broccoli florets, chopped

- 1 cup canned black beans, no-salt-added, drained
- 1 cup brown rice
- 2 cups low-sodium chicken stock
- 2 teaspoons sweet paprika
- Black pepper to taste

Preparation:
1. Put the stock in a pot, heat up over medium heat, add the rice and the other ingredients.
2. Toss, bring to a boil and cook for 30 minutes stirring from time to time.
3. Divide the mix between plates and serve as a side dish.

Serving Suggestion: Garnish with parsley.
Variation Tip: Add chili for a spicier taste.
Nutritional Information per Serving:
Calories 347 | Fat 1.2g | Sodium 83mg | Carbs 69.3g | Fiber 9g | Sugar 1.5g | Protein 15.1g

Artichokes a la Romana

Prep Time: 10 minutes
Cook Time: 55 minutes
Serves: 4
Ingredients:
- 2 cups fresh breadcrumbs
- 1 tablespoon olive oil
- 4 large globe artichokes, cored
- 2 lemons, halved and juiced
- ⅓ cup parmesan cheese, grated
- 3 garlic cloves, chopped
- 2 tablespoons fresh flat-leaf (Italian) parsley, chopped
- 1 tablespoon grated lemon zest
- ¼ teaspoon black pepper
- 1 cup and 4 tablespoons low-sodium vegetable stock
- 1 cup dry white wine
- 1 tablespoon shallot, minced
- 1 teaspoon oregano, chopped

Preparation:
1. Preheat the oven to 400°F.
2. Toss the breadcrumbs with the olive oil.
3. Spread the crumbs in a shallow baking tray.
4. Bake for 10 minutes until golden.
5. Drizzle the lemon juice over the trimmed artichokes.
6. Mix the breadcrumbs with the garlic, parmesan, lemon zest, parsley, and pepper.
7. Stir in 4 tablespoons of stock, mixing until the crumbs are clump-free.
8. Stuff the artichokes with the garlic mixture.
9. Mix 1 cup of the stock with the shallots, white wine, and oregano in a Dutch oven.

10. Bring this mixture to a boil, then decrease the heat to low.
11. Place the artichokes in the Dutch oven and cover with its lid.
12. Cook the artichokes for 45 minutes on low heat.
13. Slice the artichokes and serve.

Serving Suggestion: Serve with garlic mayo on the side.
Variation Tip: Add chopped spinach to the filling.
Nutritional Information per Serving:
Calories 123 | Fat 1g | Sodium 36mg | Carbs 17.1g | Fiber 0.3g | Sugar 0.1g | Protein 4.2g

Peanut Butter Hummus

Prep Time: 5 minutes
Cook Time: 5 minutes
Serves: 16
Ingredients
- 2 cups garbanzo beans
- 1 cup water
- ½ cup powdered peanut butter
- ¼ cup natural peanut butter
- 2 tbsp. brown sugar
- 1 tsp. vanilla extract

Preparation
1. Place all of the ingredients in a food processor. Process until smooth.
2. Refrigerate for up to 1 week.

Serving Suggestion: This fresh spin on traditional hummus can be spread on sandwiches or served as a dip for apples and celery.
Variation Tip: Add more spices, if desired.
Nutritional Information Per Serving:
Calories 135 | Protein 7g | Carbohydrate 19g | Dietary fiber 4g | Sugars 4g | Fat 4g | Sodium 47 mg

Braised Cabbage

Prep Time: 5 minutes
Cook Time: 30 minutes
Serves: 1
Ingredients:
- 1 garlic clove, minced
- 1½ cup green cabbage, chopped
- ¾ teaspoon olive oil
- ½ cup low-sodium vegetable broth
- ½ onion, sliced thinly
- Fresh ground black pepper to taste

Preparation:
1. Take a large frying pan, heat oil over medium-high heat and fry garlic for about a minute.
2. Add onion and fry for about four to five minutes.
3. Add cabbage and fry for about three to four minutes.
4. Stir in broth and black pepper and immediately, reduce the heat to low.
5. Cook while covered for about 20 minutes.
6. Serve warm and enjoy!
Serving Suggestions: Serve it with freshly chopped herbs.
Variation Tip: Season the cabbage to taste with additional salt.
Nutritional Information per Serving:
Calories: 90 | Fat: 3.7g | Sat Fat: 0.5g |
Carbohydrates: 12.8g | Fiber: 3.9g | Sugar: 5.7g | Protein: 3.2g

Lemony Zucchini

Prep Time: 15 minutes
Cook Time: 7 minutes
Serves: 6
Ingredients:
- 4 large zucchinis, sliced
- 2 tablespoons fresh lemon juice
- 2 teaspoons fresh mint leaves, minced
- 2 tablespoons canola oil
- 2 garlic cloves, minced
- Fresh ground black pepper to taste

Preparation:
1. Take a large frying pan, heat oil over medium-high heat and stir fry the zucchini and garlic for about two to three minutes.
2. Add lemon juice and black pepper and stir fry for about two minutes.
3. Stir in mint and cook for about one to two minutes.
4. Serve hot.
Serving Suggestions: Serve with coriander on top.
Variation Tip: You can also use a small amount garlic powder.
Nutritional Information per Serving:
Calories: 79 | Fat: 5.1g | Sat Fat: 0.5g|
Carbohydrates: 7.7g | Fiber: 2.5g | Sugar: 3.9g |
Protein: 2.7g

Mashed Sweet Potatoes

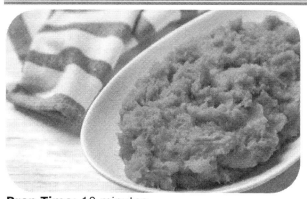

Prep Time: 10 minutes
Cook Time: 25 minutes
Serves: 4
Ingredients:
- 6 medium sweet potatoes, peeled and cubed
- 2 tablespoons unsalted butter
- ¼ cup non-fat plain Greek yogurt
- 1 teaspoon freshly ground black pepper
- ¼ teaspoon salt
- ⅓ cup milk
- ¼ cup thinly sliced scallions
- ¼ cup finely chopped fresh parsley
- 1 garlic clove, minced

Preparation:
1. In a large saucepan, combine the sweet potatoes and enough water to cover them by 1 inch.
2. Bring to a boil, then reduce the heat to a simmer and cook for 10 to 15 minutes, or until the sweet potatoes are tender.
3. Drain well and return the sweet potatoes to the saucepan. Add the butter, yogurt, pepper and salt.
4. Using a hand mixer, a potato masher, or a fork, blend while slowly adding the milk until the ingredients are mixed.
5. Add the scallions, parsley, and garlic and mix until well combined. Let cool, then serve.
Serving Suggestion: Serve with baked Tilapia or turkey breast.
Variation Tip: To save time and effort, you can purchase frozen sweet potato cubes.
Nutritional Information per Serving:
Calories 242 | Fat 6g | Sodium 271mg | Carbs 42g |
Fiber 6.5g | Sugar 14g | Protein 6g

Broccoli with Bell Peppers

Prep Time: 5 minutes
Cook Time: 10 minutes
Serves: 3
Ingredients:
- 1 garlic clove, minced
- 1½ large bell peppers, seeded and sliced
- 2 tablespoons low-sodium vegetable broth
- 1 cup small broccoli florets
- ½ large yellow onion, sliced
- 1 tablespoon olive oil
- Fresh ground black pepper to taste

Preparation:
1. In a large frying-pan, heat the oil over medium heat and fry the garlic for about a minute.
2. Add the vegetables and stir fry for about five minutes.
3. Stir in the broth and soy sauce and stir fry for about four minutes.
4. Stir in the black pepper and remove from the heat.
5. Serve hot and enjoy!

Serving Suggestions: Serve with roasted sesame seeds on top.
Variation Tip: You can spice it up a little bit using red pepper flakes.
Nutritional Information per Serving:
Calories: 78 | Fat: 4.9g | Sat Fat: 0.7g | Carbohydrates: 8.5g | Fiber: 1.4g | Sugar: 4.1g | Protein: 1.7g

Coconut Shrimp

Prep Time: 20 minutes
Cook Time: 10 minutes
Serves: 6
Ingredients
- ¼ cup sweetened coconut
- ¼ cup panko breadcrumbs
- ½ tsp. kosher salt
- ½ cup coconut milk
- 12 large shrimp, peeled and deveined

Preparation
1. Heat the oven to 375°F. Lightly coat a baking sheet with cooking spray.
2. Place the coconut, panko, and salt in a food processor and process until the mixture is an even consistency. Place the panko mixture in a small bowl.
3. Place the coconut milk in another small bowl. Dip each shrimp in the coconut milk and then in the panko mixture, and place on the baking sheet.
4. Lightly coat the top of the shrimp with cooking spray. Bake until golden brown (about 10 to 15 minutes).

Serving Suggestion: Serve hot.
Variation Tip: You can use smaller shrimp. Just plan for less breading and less baking time.
Nutritional Information Per Serving:
Calories 75 | Protein 5g | Carbohydrate 4g | Dietary fiber 0g | Sugars 2g | Fat 4g | Sodium 396mg

Chipotle Spiced Shrimp

Prep Time: 45 minutes
Cook Time: 5 minutes
Serves: 4
Ingredients
- 1 lb. uncooked shrimp, peeled and deveined
- 2 tbsp. tomato paste
- 1½ tsp. water
- ½ tsp. extra-virgin olive oil
- ½ tsp. minced garlic
- ½ tsp. chipotle chili powder
- ½ tsp. chopped fresh oregano

Preparation
1. Rinse the shrimp in cold water. Pat dry with a paper towel and set aside on a plate.
2. To make the marinade, whisk together the tomato paste, water, and oil in a small bowl. Add the garlic, chili powder, and oregano. Mix well.
3. Using a brush, spread the marinade (it will be thick) on both sides of the shrimp. Place the marinated shrimp in the refrigerator.
4. Prepare a hot fire in a charcoal grill or heat a broiler. Away from the heat source, lightly coat the grill rack or broiler pan with cooking spray. Position the cooking rack 4 to 6 inches from the heat source.
5. Put the shrimp in a grill basket or on skewers and place it on the grill. Turn the shrimp after 3 to 4 minutes. The cooking time varies depending on the heat of the fire, so watch carefully.

Serving Suggestion: Transfer to a plate and serve immediately.
Variation Tip: Add spices of your choice.
Nutritional Information Per Serving:
Calories 109 | Protein 23g | Carbohydrate 2g | Dietary fiber 0.5g | Sugar 0g | Fat 1g | Sodium 139mg

Lemony Mushrooms

Prep Time: 5 minutes
Cook Time: 11 minutes
Serves: 1
Ingredients:
- ¼ cup shallots, chopped
- 1 teaspoon olive oil
- 1½ cups fresh oyster mushrooms, sliced
- 1 tablespoon fresh lemon juice
- Fresh ground black pepper to taste

Preparation:
1. Take a large skillet, heat oil over medium heat and fry the shallot for about two to three minutes.
2. Add mushrooms and black pepper and cook for about five to seven minutes or until mushrooms become tender.
3. Stir in lemon juice and remove from heat.
4. Serve immediately enjoy!

Serving Suggestions: Serve with lemon on side and garnish with parsley.
Variation Tip: Try to use sliced mushrooms.
Nutritional Information per Serving:
Calories: 110 | Fat: 4.8g | Sat Fat: 0.8g |
Carbohydrates: 13.1g | Fiber: 1.2g | Sugar: 0.3g |
Protein: 4.1g

Baked Brie Envelopes

Prep Time: 15 minutes
Cook Time: 22 minutes
Serves: 4
Ingredients:
- ½ cup fresh cranberries
- 2 tablespoons sugar
- ½ medium orange, quartered
- 1 cinnamon stick
- 6 ounces Brie cheese, cut into ½-ounce cubes
- 1 sheet puff pastry dough, sliced into 12 squares
- 2 tablespoons water
- 1 egg white

Preparation:
1. Preheat the oven to 425°F.
2. Grease a small sauté pan and heat it.
3. Add the orange, cranberries, sugar, and cinnamon stick.
4. Sauté for 10 minutes until the mixture thickens.
5. Remove the orange and the cinnamon sticks from the sauce.
6. Add one cube of cheese and 1 teaspoon of cooled cranberry to each of the puff pastry squares.
7. Beat the egg white with the water and dab the edges of the puff pastry with this mixture.
8. Fold the edges of the pastry squares and seal them to create envelopes.
9. Brush each envelope with the remaining egg wash.
10. Place the envelopes on a baking sheet and bake for 12 minutes.
11. Serve.

Serving Suggestion: Serve with apple sauce on the side.
Variation Tip: Add chopped apples to the brie filling.
Nutritional Information per Serving:
Calories 116 | Fat 7g |Sodium 50mg | Carbs 38g |
Fiber 6.3g | Sugar 1g | Protein 4 g

Pesto Stuffed Mushrooms

Prep Time: 15 minutes
Cook Time: 15 minutes
Serves: 10
Ingredients:
- 20 cremini mushrooms, stemmed
Topping:
- 1½ cups panko breadcrumbs
- ¼ cup melted butter
- 3 tablespoons fresh parsley, chopped
Filling:
- 2 cups fresh basil leaves
- ¼ cup fresh parmesan cheese
- 2 tablespoons pumpkin seeds
- 1 tablespoon olive oil
- 1 tablespoon fresh garlic
- 2 teaspoons lemon juice
- ½ teaspoon kosher salt

Preparation:
1. Preheat the oven to 350°F.
2. Arrange the mushroom caps upside down on a baking sheet.
3. Prepare the topping by mixing the panko, parsley, and butter in a bowl.

4. Mix the basil, pumpkin seeds, cheese, garlic, oil, and lemon juice in a blender. Blend well.
5. Stuff the mushroom caps with the basil paste and top them with the panko mixture.
6. Press the mixture into the caps.
7. Bake for 15 minutes until golden brown.
8. Serve.
Serving Suggestion: Serve with chili sauce on the side.
Variation Tip: Use coleslaw to top the mushrooms.
Nutritional Information per Serving:
Calories 159 | Fat 3g |Sodium 63mg | Carbs 4g | Fiber 0.3g | Sugar 0.3g | Protein 2g

Artichokes al la Romana

Prep Time: 20 minutes
Cook Time: 45 minutes
Serves: 8
Ingredients
• 2 cups fresh breadcrumbs, preferably whole-wheat
• 1 tbsp. olive oil
• 4 large globe artichokes
• 2 lemons, halved
• ⅓ cup grated parmesan cheese
• 3 garlic cloves, finely chopped
• 2 tbsp. finely chopped fresh flat-leaf (Italian) parsley
• 1 tbsp. grated lemon zest
• ¼ tsp. freshly ground black pepper
• 1 cup plus 2 to 4 tbsp. low-sodium vegetable or chicken stock
• 1 cup dry white wine
• 1 tbsp. minced shallot
• 1 tsp. chopped fresh oregano
Preparation
1. Heat the oven to 400°F. In a bowl, combine the breadcrumbs and olive oil. Toss to coat. Spread the crumbs in a shallow baking pan and bake, stirring once halfway through, until the crumbs are lightly golden (about 10 minutes). Set aside to cool.
2. Working with 1 artichoke at a time, snap off any tough outer leaves and trim the stem flush with the base. Cut off the top third of the leaves with a serrated knife, and trim off any remaining thorns with scissors. Rub the cut edges with a lemon half to prevent discoloration. Separate the inner leaves and pull out the small leaves from the center. Using a melon baller or spoon, scoop out the fuzzy choke, then squeeze some lemon juice into the cavity. Trim the remaining artichokes in the same manner.

3. Toss the breadcrumbs with the parmesan, garlic, parsley, lemon zest, and pepper in a large bowl. Add the 2 to 4 tbsp. stock, 1 tbsp. at a time. Use just enough for the stuffing to begin to stick together in small clumps.
4. Using 2/3 of the stuffing, mound it slightly in the center of the artichokes. Then, starting at the bottom, spread the leaves open and spoon a rounded teaspoon of stuffing near the base of each leaf. (The artichokes can be prepared to this point several hours ahead and kept refrigerated.)
5. In a Dutch oven with a tight-fitting lid, combine the 1 cup stock, wine, shallot, and oregano. (Note: Don't use cast iron, or the cooked artichokes will turn brown.) Bring to a boil, then reduce the heat to low. Arrange the artichokes, stem-end down, in the liquid in a single layer. Cover and simmer until the outer leaves are tender (about 45 minutes, add water if necessary).
Serving Suggestion: Transfer the artichokes to a rack and let cool slightly. Cut each artichoke into quarters and serve warm.
Variation Tip: Add spices of your choice.
Nutritional Information Per Serving:
Calories 123 | Protein 6g | Carbohydrate 18g | Dietary fiber 5g | Sugar 0g | Fat 3g | Sodium 179mg

Rosemary Potato Shells

Prep Time: 15 minutes
Cook Time: 1 hour and 5 minutes
Serves: 4
Ingredients:
• 2 medium russet potatoes
• Butter-flavored cooking spray
• 1 tablespoon fresh rosemary, finely chopped
• ⅛ teaspoon black pepper
Preparation:
1. Preheat the oven to 375°F.
2. Pierce the mashed potatoes with a fork and place them on a baking sheet.
3. Bake for 1 hour until crispy.
4. Allow the potatoes to cool before handling, then cut them in half.
5. Scoop out the pulp, leaving the ⅛-inch-thick shell.
6. Coat the shells with the butter-flavored cooking spray and season with the pepper and rosemary.
7. Bake for another 5 minutes.
8. Serve.
Serving Suggestion: Serve with tomato sauce on the side.
Variation Tip: Add mixed dried herbs on top.
Nutritional Information per Serving:
Calories 167 | Fat 0g |Sodium 119mg | Carbs 27g | Fiber 0.5g | Sugar 1.4g | Protein 7.8g

Tomato Basil Bruschetta

Prep Time: 30 minutes
Cook Time: 10 minutes
Serves: 6
Ingredients
- ½ whole-grain baguette, cut into six ½-inch-thick diagonal slices
- 2 tbsp. chopped basil
- 1 tbsp. chopped parsley
- 2 cloves garlic, minced
- 3 tomatoes, diced
- ½ cup diced fennel
- 1 tsp. olive oil
- 2 tsp. balsamic vinegar
- 1 tsp. black pepper

Preparation
1. Heat the oven to 400°F. Toast the baguette slices in the oven until lightly browned.
2. Meanwhile, mix all the other ingredients together.
3. Spoon the mixture evenly over the toasted bread.
Serving Suggestion: Serve immediately.
Variation Tip: If you want a drier topping, remove the seeds from the tomato before dicing. (Cut the tomatoes in half and scoop out the seeds with your finger or a spoon.)
Nutritional Information Per Serving:
Calories 142 | Protein 5g | Carbohydrate 26g | Dietary fiber 4g | Sugars 0g | Fat 2g | Sodium 123mg

Basil Tomato Crostini

Prep Time: 10 minutes
Cook Time: 0 minutes
Serves: 2
Ingredients:

- 4 plum tomatoes, chopped
- ¼ cup minced fresh basil
- 2 teaspoons olive oil
- 1 garlic clove, minced
- Freshly ground pepper
- ¼ pound Italian bread, cut into 4 slices and toasted

Preparation:
1. Toss the tomatoes with the oil, garlic, pepper, and basil in a bowl.
2. Cover and allow them to sit for 30 minutes.
3. Top the toast slices with the mixture.
4. Serve.
Serving Suggestion: Serve with a sprinkling of chopped herbs on top.
Variation Tip: Add paprika more spice.
Nutritional Information per Serving:
Calories 104 | Fat 3.5g |Sodium 53mg | Carbs 15g | Fiber 0.4g | Sugar 1g | Protein 2g

Marinated Portobello Mushrooms with Provolone

Prep Time: 20 minutes
Cook Time: 20 minutes
Serves: 2
Ingredients
- 2 portobello mushrooms, stemmed and wiped clean
- ½ cup balsamic vinegar
- 1 tbsp. brown sugar
- ¼ tsp. dried rosemary
- 1 tsp. minced garlic
- ¼ cup grated (1 oz.) provolone cheese

Preparation
1. Heat the broiler. Position the rack 4 inches from the heat source. Lightly coat a glass baking dish with cooking spray. Place the mushrooms in the dish, stemless-side (gill-side) up.
2. In a small bowl, whisk together the vinegar, brown sugar, rosemary, and garlic. Pour the mixture over the mushrooms. Set aside for 5 to 10 minutes to marinate.
3. Broil the mushrooms, turning once, until tender (about 4 minutes on each side).
Serving Suggestion: Sprinkle grated cheese over each mushroom and continue to broil until the cheese melts. Transfer to individual plates.
Variation Tip: Add spices or herbs of your choice.
Nutritional Information Per Serving:
Calories 112 | Protein 6g | Carbohydrate 13g | Dietary fiber 1g | Sugars 4g | Fat 4g | Sodium 140mg

Butternut Squash Fries

Prep Time: 10 minutes
Cook Time: 15 minutes
Serves: 4
Ingredients:
- 1 medium butternut squash
- 1 tablespoon olive oil
- 1 tablespoon fresh thyme, chopped
- 1 tablespoon fresh rosemary, chopped
- ½ teaspoon salt

Preparation:
1. Preheat the oven to 425°F.
2. Grease a baking sheet with cooking spray.
3. Peel the squash and slice it into 3-inch-long and ½-inch wide pieces.
4. Place the pieces in a large bowl and toss with the oil, thyme, salt, and rosemary.
5. Spread the squash on the baking sheet and bake for 10 minutes.
6. Toss the fries well and bake again for 5 minutes or more until golden brown.
7. Serve.

Serving Suggestion: Serve with tomato sauce on the side.
Variation Tip: Add lemon juice and lemon zest on top.
Nutritional Information per Serving:
Calories 117 | Fat 19g |Sodium 57mg | Carbs 29g | Fiber 1.8g | Sugar 1.2g | Protein 2.5g

Zucchini Pizza Bites

Prep Time: 10 minutes
Cook Time: 4 minutes
Serves: 4

Ingredients:
- 4 slices large zucchini, cut ¼-inch thick
- Olive oil spray
- Black pepper, to taste
- 4 tablespoons pizza sauce
- 2 tablespoons part-skim mozzarella cheese, shredded

Preparation:
1. Preheat the broiler on high.
2. Season the zucchini slices with the pepper and olive oil.
3. Place the slices on a baking sheet and broil them for 2 minutes.
4. Top each zucchini slice with pizza sauce and cheese.
5. Broil for another 2 minutes.
6. Serve warm.

Serving Suggestion: Serve with tomato sauce on the side.
Variation Tip: Replace the zucchini slices with eggplant slices
Nutritional Information per Serving:
Calories 192 | Fat 6g |Sodium 66mg | Carbs 39g | Fiber 0.9g | Sugar 0.6g | Protein 8g

Smoked Trout Spread

Prep Time: 15 minutes
Cook Time: 0 minutes
Serves: 6
Ingredients:
- ¼ pound smoked trout fillet, skinned and broken into pieces
- ½ cup 1% low-fat cottage cheese
- ¼ cup red onion, coarsely chopped
- 2 teaspoons fresh lemon juice
- 1 teaspoon hot pepper sauce
- ½ teaspoon Worcestershire sauce
- 1 celery stalk, diced

Preparation:
1. Blend the trout with the cottage cheese, lemon juice, Worcestershire sauce, red onion, and hot pepper sauce in a food processor.
2. Continue blending until smooth.
3. Fold in the diced celery, then cover the spread.
4. Refrigerate and serve.

Serving Suggestion: Serve with celery sticks on the side.
Variation Tip: Drizzle lemon juice on top before serving.
Nutritional Information per Serving:
Calories 201 | Fat 24.5g |Sodium 34mg | Carbs 9.3g | Fiber 1.4g | Sugar 1g | Protein 3g

Black Bean Dip

Prep Time: 10 minutes
Cook Time: 2 minutes
Serves: 2
Ingredients:
• 1 (15 ounces) can black beans, drained, with liquid reserved
• ½ (7 ounces) can Chipotle peppers in Adobo sauce
• ¼ cup plain Greek yogurt
• Black pepper, to taste
Preparation:
1. Combine beans, peppers, and yogurt in a food processor or blender and process until smooth.
2. Add some of the bean liquid, 1 tablespoon at a time, for a thinner consistency.
3. Season to taste with black pepper.
4. Serve.
Serving Suggestion: Garnish with basil leaves.
Variation Tip: As an alternative, you could use 1 teaspoon dry chipotle chili powder.
Nutritional Information per Serving:
Calories 70 | Fat 1 g | Sodium 159 mg | Carbs 11 g | Fiber4 g | Sugar 0 g | Protein 5 g

Crispy Garbanzo Beans

Prep Time: 15 minutes
Cook Time: 40 minutes
Serves: 6
Ingredients:
• 2 cans (15 ounces each) unsalted garbanzo beans
• ½ teaspoon salt
• ½ teaspoon pepper
• 1 teaspoon garlic powder
• 1 teaspoon onion powder
• 1 teaspoon dried parsley flakes
• 2 teaspoon dried dill

• Cooking spray
Preparation:
1. Preheat the oven to 400°F.
2. Rinse and drain all the garbanzo beans. Absorb all the excess water out of them.
3. Mix all the remaining ingredients in a bowl.
4. Toss in the garbanzo beans and mix well to coat.
5. Spread the beans on a greased baking sheet.
6. Place the baking sheet on the lowest rack of the oven.
7. Roast the beans for about 30 to 40 minutes until golden brown.
8. Give them a gentle stir every 15 minutes.
9. Serve.
Serving Suggestion: Serve with roasted nuts.
Variation Tip: Add cinnamon powder on top.
Nutritional Information per Serving:
Calories 218 | Fat 4.7g |Sodium 994mg | Carbs 31.9g | Fiber 0.4g | Sugar 3g | Protein 5.6g

Sweet Snack Mix

Prep Time: 10 minutes
Cook Time: 45 minutes
Serves: 6
Ingredients:
• 2 cans (15 ounces each) garbanzo beans, drained
• 2 cups wheat squares cereal
• 1 cup dried pineapple chunks
• 1 cup raisins
• 2 tablespoons honey
• 2 tablespoons Worcestershire sauce
• 1 teaspoon garlic powder
• ½ teaspoon chili powder
Preparation:
1. Preheat the oven to 350°F. Grease a baking sheet with butter spray.
2. Grease a skillet with cooking spray and sauté the beans in it for 10 minutes.
3. Transfer the beans to the baking sheet and bake for 20 minutes.
4. Toss the raisins, cereal, and pineapple into the beans.
5. Combine the spices with the honey and Worcestershire sauce in a bowl.
6. Pour this sauce over the beans.
7. Mix well and bake the beans again for 15 minutes, stirring occasionally.
8. Serve.
Serving Suggestion: Serve with apple sauce on top.
Variation Tip: You can replace the raisins with cranberries.
Nutritional Information per Serving:
Calories 209 | Fat 7g |Sodium 26mg | Carbs 34g | Fiber 0.3g | Sugar 0.3g | Protein 3g

Parsley Mushrooms

Prep Time: 5 minutes
Cook Time: 14 minutes
Serves: 1

Ingredients:
- 1-2 tablespoon onion, minced
- 6 ounces fresh mushrooms, sliced
- ½ tablespoon fresh parsley, chopped
- 1 tablespoon olive oil
- ½ teaspoon garlic, minced
- Pinch of salt
- Fresh ground black pepper to taste

Preparation:
1. In a frying-pan, heat the oil over medium heat and fry the onion and garlic for two to three minutes.
2. Add the mushrooms and cook for eight to ten minutes.
3. Stir in the parsley salt and black pepper and remove from the heat.
4. Serve hot and enjoy!

Serving Suggestions: Serve with chopped parsley as a topping.
Variation Tip: If you are using fine salt, add only a little amount.
Nutritional Information per Serving:
Calories: 163 | Fat: 14.5g | Sat Fat: 2g | Carbohydrates: 7.2g | Fiber: 2g | Sugar: 3.4g | Protein: 5.6g

Zucchini and Brussels Sprouts Salad

Prep Time: 10 minutes
Cook Time: 3 hours
Serves: 4
Ingredients:
- 1-pound zucchinis, roughly cubed
- ½ pound Brussels sprouts, trimmed and halved
- ¼ cup veggie stock, low-sodium
- 1 teaspoon cumin, ground
- 1 teaspoon chili powder
- 2 teaspoon avocado oil

Preparation:
1. In a slow cooker, mix the sprouts with zucchini and other ingredients.
2. Cover, and simmer for 3 hours on low.
3. Divide between plates and serve as a side dish.
Serving Suggestion: Top with pine nuts.
Variation Tip: Substitute avocado oil with olive oil.
Nutritional Information per Serving:
Calories 51 | Fat 0.9 g | Sodium 42 mg | Carbs 9.8 g | Fiber 3.8 g | Sugar 3.3 g | Protein 3.5 g

Pickled Asparagus

Prep Time: 10 minutes
Cook Time: 0 minutes
Serves: 6
Ingredients:
- 3 cups fresh asparagus, trimmed
- ¼ cup pearl onions
- ¼ cup white wine vinegar
- ¼ cup cider vinegar
- 1 sprig fresh dill
- 1 cup water
- 2 whole cloves
- 3 garlic cloves, whole
- 8 whole black peppercorns
- ¼ teaspoon red pepper flakes
- 6 whole coriander seeds

Preparation:
1. Trim and cut the asparagus spears into jar size pieces.
2. Place these spears in a colander and rinse them.
3. Put the asparagus with the trimmed onions into a large mason jar.
4. Add all the other ingredients and seal the jar.
5. Refrigerate for 4 weeks.
6. Serve.
Serving Suggestion: Serve with cheese dip on the side.
Variation Tip: Add minced jalapenos to the pickling juices.
Nutritional Information per Serving:
Calories 76 | Fat 1g |Sodium 27mg | Carbs 4g | Fiber 1g | Sugar 3g | Protein 2g

Chili-Lime Grilled Pineapple

Prep Time: 5 minutes
Cook Time: 15 minutes
Servings: 6
Ingredients:
- 1 fresh pineapple
- 3 tablespoons brown sugar
- 1 tablespoon lime juice
- 1 tablespoon olive oil
- 1 tablespoon honey
- 1½ teaspoons chili powder
- Dash of salt

Preparation:
1. Peel the pineapple. Remove the core and cut the fruit lengthwise into six wedges.
2. Mix the remaining ingredients in a small bowl until well combined. Brush the pineapple wedges with half of the glaze; reserve the remaining mixture for basting.
3. Grill the pineapple wedges for 2–4 minutes on each side over medium heat or broil 4 inches from the heat source until nicely browned, occasionally basting with the leftover glaze.
4. Serve and enjoy!

Serving Suggestion: Serve with steak.
Variation Tip: You can use agave nectar instead of honey.
Nutritional Information per Serving:
Calories: 97|Fat: 2g|Sat Fat: 0g|Carbohydrates: 50g|Fiber: 1g|Sugar: 13g|Protein: 1g

Apple Nachos

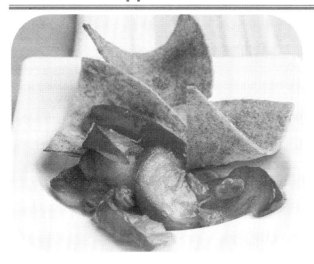

Prep Time: 10 minutes
Cook Time: 10 minutes
Serves: 6
Ingredients:
- ½ teaspoon apple pie spice
- Non-stick cooking spray
- 1 teaspoon granulated sugar
- 2 apples, cored and sliced
- 2 (6 or 7-inch) wheat tortillas
- ½ cup water
- 1 tablespoon brown sugar
- 1 tablespoon golden raisins
- ½ teaspoon orange peel, finely shredded

Preparation:
1. Preheat the oven to 400°F.
2. Coat both sides of the tortillas with non-stick cooking spray.
3. Dice each tortilla into 6 wedges.
4. Mix them with the apple pie spice and sugar in a bowl.
5. Spread the tortilla wedges on a baking sheet and bake for 10 minutes.
6. Meanwhile, mix all the remaining ingredients in a saucepan.
7. Let the sauce boil, then reduce the heat.
8. Let it cool for about 10 minutes.

Serving Suggestion: Serve with maple syrup or applesauce on the side.
Variation Tip: Add whipping cream on top.
Nutritional Information per Serving:
Calories 219 | Fat 6.4g |Sodium 46mg | Carbs 30.4g | Fiber 0.1g | Sugar 10.4g | Protein 8.5g

Pickled Eggs

Prep Time: 15 minutes
Cook Time: 15 minutes
Serves: 6
Ingredients:
- 15 ounces beets liquid
- 1 cup cider vinegar
- ½ cup sugar
- 2 bay leaves
- 4 whole cloves
- 1 onion, sliced into rings
- 6 large eggs

Preparation:

1. Mix the beets liquid with the cloves, bay leaves, sugar, and vinegar in a saucepan.
2. Bring the mixture to a boil and mix well to dissolve the sugar.
3. Pour this liquid into a deep bowl.
4. Add the onions to the liquid and set it aside for 1 hour.
5. Place the eggs in a saucepan and cover them with water.
6. Bring to a boil, then reduce the heat to simmer. Cook for 10 minutes.
7. Drain and rinse the eggs under cold water.
8. Peel each egg and transfer them to the onion liquid.
9. Cover the bowl and refrigerate for 24 hours.
10. Drain the eggs and slice them in half.
11. Serve.

Serving Suggestion: Serve with avocado sauce on the side.

Variation Tip: Add chopped chives on top of the eggs.

Nutritional Information per Serving:
Calories 121 | Fat 7.4g |Sodium 56mg | Carbs 23g | Fiber 2.4g | Sugar 5g | Protein 13.2g

Braised Bell Peppers

Prep Time: 15 minutes
Cook Time: 10 minutes
Serves: 6
Ingredients:
• 1 cup onion, sliced
• 3 teaspoons garlic, minced
• 2 tablespoons canola oil
• 8 cups bell peppers, seeded and julienned
• ½ cup low-sodium vegetable broth
• Fresh ground black pepper to taste
Preparation:
1. Take a large frying pan, heat oil over medium-high heat and fry onion and bell peppers for about four to five minutes.
2. Add garlic and fry for about a minute.
3. Add the remaining ingredients and stir to combine well.
4. Reduce the heat to medium and cook for about three to four minutes, stirring occasionally.
5. Serve hot.
Serving Suggestions: Sere it with pizza as a topping.
Variation Tip: Stir in black pepper and vinegar for better taste.
Nutritional Information per Serving:

Calories: 103 | Fat: 5.1g | Sat Fat: 0.3g | Carbohydrates: 14.3g | Fiber: 2.6g | Sugar: 8.8g | Protein: 2.1g

Sausage-Stuffed Zucchini

Prep Time: 35 minutes
Cook Time: 20 minutes
Servings: 6
Ingredients:
• 6 medium zucchinis
• 1 pound Italian turkey sausage links, casings removed
• 2 medium tomatoes, seeded and chopped
• 1 cup panko breadcrumbs
• ⅓ cup parmesan cheese, grated
• ⅓ cup fresh parsley, minced
• 2 tablespoons fresh oregano, minced
• 2 tablespoons fresh basil, minced
• ¼ teaspoon pepper
• ¾ cup part-skim mozzarella cheese, shredded
Preparation:
1. Preheat the oven to 350°F. Cut each zucchini in half lengthwise. Scoop out the pulp, leaving a ¼-inch shell. Set the pulp aside.
2. Place the zucchini in batches in a large microwave-safe dish, cover, and microwave on high power for 2–3 minutes or until crisp-tender.
3. Cook the sausage and zucchini pulp in a large skillet over medium heat for 6–8 minutes, or until the meat is no longer pink. Ensure that the sausage meat is broken into crumbs; drain.
4. Combine the tomatoes, breadcrumbs, parmesan cheese, herbs, and pepper in a mixing bowl. Fill the zucchini shells with the mixture.
5. Place in two 13-inch x 9-inch baking dishes. Cook for 15–20 minutes, covered, or until the zucchini is soft.
6. Sprinkle with the mozzarella cheese. Bake for another 5–8 minutes, uncovered, or until the cheese has melted.
7. Serve and enjoy!
Serving Suggestion: Sprinkle with additional minced parsley.
Variation Tip: You can use dried oregano instead of freshly minced oregano.
Nutritional Information per Serving:
Calories: 206|Fat: 9g|Sat Fat: 3g|Carbohydrates: 16g|Fiber: 3g|Sugar: 5g|Protein: 17g

Cannellini Bean Hummus

Prep Time: 5 minutes
Cook Time: 5 minutes
Servings: 10
Ingredients:
- 2 garlic cloves, peeled
- 1 can cannellini beans, rinsed and drained
- ¼ cup tahini
- 3 tablespoons lemon juice
- 1½ teaspoons ground cumin
- ¼ teaspoon salt
- ¼ teaspoon crushed red pepper flakes
- 2 tablespoons fresh parsley, minced

Preparation:
1. Pulse the garlic in a food processor until minced. Add the beans, tahini, lemon juice, cumin, salt, and pepper flakes and pulse until smooth.
2. Transfer the mixture to a small mixing dish and add the parsley. Refrigerate until ready to serve.
3. Serve and enjoy!

Serving Suggestion: Serve with pita bread wedges.
Variation Tip: You can also serve with assorted fresh vegetables.
Nutritional Information per Serving:
Calories: 78|Fat: 4g|Sat Fat: 1g|Carbohydrates: 8g|Fiber: 2g|Sugar: 0g|Protein: 3g

Portobello Mushroom Florentine

Prep Time: 5 minutes

Cook Time: 25 minutes
Servings: 2
Ingredients:
- 2 large portobello mushrooms, stems removed
- Cooking spray
- ⅛ teaspoon garlic salt
- ⅛ teaspoon pepper
- ½ teaspoon olive oil
- 1 small onion, chopped
- 1 cup fresh baby spinach
- 2 large eggs
- ⅛ teaspoon salt

Preparation:
1. Preheat the oven to 425°F. Spritz the mushrooms with cooking spray and lay them stem side up on a baking sheet.
2. Add garlic salt and pepper to taste. Bake the mushrooms in the preheated oven for about 10 minutes.
3. Meanwhile, heat the oil in a non-stick skillet over medium-high heat and cook the onion until tender. Stir in the spinach and cook until it's completely wilted.
4. Whisk together the eggs and salt and pour the mixture into the skillet. Cook, constantly stirring, until the eggs have thickened and there's no liquid egg left. Spoon the mixture over the cooked mushrooms.
5. Serve and enjoy!

Serving Suggestion: Sprinkle with basil.
Variation Tip: You can also top with feta cheese.
Nutritional Information per Serving:
Calories: 126|Fat: 5g|Sat Fat: 2g|Carbohydrates: 10g|Fiber: 3g|Sugar: 4g|Protein: 11g

Cherry-Chicken Lettuce Wraps

Prep Time: 5 minutes
Cook Time: 25 minutes
Servings: 4
Ingredients:
- ¾ pound boneless, skinless chicken breasts, cut into cubes
- 1 teaspoon ground ginger
- ¼ teaspoon salt
- ¼ teaspoon pepper
- 2 teaspoons olive oil
- 1½ cups carrots, shredded
- 1¼ cups pitted fresh sweet cherries, coarsely chopped
- 4 green onions, chopped
- 2 tablespoons rice vinegar
- 2 tablespoons reduced-sodium teriyaki sauce

- 1 tablespoon honey
- 8 Bibb or Boston lettuce leaves

Preparation:
1. Sprinkle the chicken with the ginger, salt, and pepper.
2. Heat the oil in a skillet and cook the chicken for 3–5 minutes, or until it's no longer pink.
3. Remove the skillet from the heat. Stir in the carrots, cherries, and green onions.
4. Combine the vinegar, teriyaki sauce, and honey in a small bowl; stir into the chicken mixture.
5. Divide the filling among the lettuce leaves and fold the lettuce over.
6. Serve and enjoy!

Serving Suggestion: Sprinkle with cilantro.
Variation Tip: You can also add coarsely chopped almonds.
Nutritional Information per Serving:
Calories: 257|Fat: 10g|Sat Fat: 1g|Carbohydrates: 22g|Fiber: 4g|Sugar: 15g|Protein: 21g

Thai-Style Cobb Salad

Prep Time: 5 minutes
Cook Time: 15 minutes
Servings: 6
Ingredients:
- 1 bunch romaine lettuce, torn
- 2 cups rotisserie chicken, shredded
- 3 large hard-boiled eggs, coarsely chopped
- 1 medium ripe avocado, peeled and thinly sliced
- 1 medium carrot, shredded
- 1 medium sweet red pepper, julienned
- 1 cup fresh snow peas, halved
- ½ cup unsalted peanuts
- ¼ cup fresh cilantro leaves
- ¾ cup Asian toasted sesame salad dressing
- 2 tablespoons creamy peanut butter

Preparation:
1. Arrange the romaine lettuce on a serving plate. Layer the chicken, eggs, avocado, veggies, and peanuts over the lettuce and; top with the cilantro.
2. Whisk the salad dressing and peanut butter together in a small bowl until smooth. Serve alongside the lettuce.
3. Serve and enjoy!

Serving Suggestion: Serve with any dish.
Variation Tip: You can also add vegetables of your choice.
Nutritional Information per Serving:
Calories: 382|Fat: 25g|Sat Fat: 5g|Carbohydrates: 18g|Fiber: 5g|Sugar: 10g|Protein: 23g

Sweet Potato and Chickpea Pitas

Prep Time: 10 minutes
Cook Time: 20 minutes
Servings: 6
Ingredients:
- 2 medium sweet potatoes, peeled and cubed
- 2 cans chickpeas or garbanzo beans, rinsed and drained
- 1 medium red onion, chopped
- 3 tablespoons canola oil, divided
- 2 teaspoons garam masala
- ½ teaspoon salt, divided
- 2 garlic cloves, minced
- 1 cup plain Greek yogurt
- 1 tablespoon lemon juice
- 1 teaspoon ground cumin
- 2 cups arugula or baby spinach
- 12 whole-wheat pita pocket halves, warmed
- ¼ cup fresh cilantro, minced

Preparation:
1. Preheat the oven to 400°F. Microwave the potatoes for 5 minutes on high power, covered, in a large microwave-safe bowl.
2. Add 2 tablespoons of oil, garam masala, and ¼ teaspoon of salt after adding the chickpeas and onion.
3. Fill a baking pan halfway with the mixture and roast in the preheated oven for 15 minutes, or until the potatoes are soft. Allow the mixture to cool slightly.
4. In a microwave-safe bowl, combine the garlic and remaining oil; microwave on high power for 1 to 1½ minutes, or until the garlic is gently browned.
5. Combine the yogurt, lemon juice, cumin, and the remaining salt in a mixing bowl.
6. Toss the arugula with the potato mixture. Fill the pitas halfway with the filling, then top with the sauce.
7. Serve and enjoy!

Serving Suggestion: Sprinkle with fresh cilantro.
Variation Tip: You can sprinkle the filling with cheese.
Nutritional Information per Serving:
Calories: 462|Fat: 15g|Sat Fat: 3g|Carbohydrates: 72g|Fiber: 12g|Sugar: 13g|Protein: 14g

Spicy Okra

Prep Time: 5 minutes
Cook Time: 12 minutes
Serves: 1
Ingredients:
• ¼ teaspoon cumin seeds
• ¼ teaspoon curry powder
• ¼ teaspoon red chili powder
• ½ tablespoon olive oil
• ⅜ pounds okra pods, trimmed and cut into 2-inch pieces
• ½ teaspoon ground coriander
Preparation:
1. In a large prying pan, heat oil over medium heat and fry cumin seeds for about 30 seconds.
2. Add okra and stir fry for about 1-1½ minutes.
3. Reduce the heat to low and cook while covered for about six to eight minutes, stirring occasionally.
4. Uncover and increase the heat to medium.
5. Stir in curry powder, red chili and coriander and cook for about two to three minutes more.
6. Serve hot and enjoy!
Serving Suggestions: Serve with lots of chopped onion.
Variation Tip: Use small organic okra when making the dish.
Nutritional Information per Serving:
Calories: 134 | Fat: 7.6g | Sat Fat: 1.1g | Carbohydrates: 13.6g | Fiber: 5.9g | Sugar: 2.6g | Protein: 3.5g

Garlicky Green Beans

Prep Time: 5 minutes

Cook Time: 11 minutes
Serves: 3
Ingredients:
• 2 garlic cloves, minced
• 1 tablespoon olive oil
• 1 pound fresh green beans, trimmed and cut-into 1-inch pieces
• Pinch of salt
• Fresh ground black pepper to taste
Preparation:
1. Take a large frying pan, heat oil over medium heat and fry garlic for about a minute.
2. Add green beans, salt and black pepper and cook for about eight to ten minutes.
3. Serve hot and enjoy!
Serving Suggestions: Serve it with your favorite snacks.
Variation Tip: Try to use real garlic instead of minced ones in a jar.
Nutritional Information per Serving:

Calories: 90 | Fat: 4.9g | Sat Fat: 0.7g | Carbohydrates: 11.5g | Fiber: 5.2g | Sugar: 2.1g | Protein: 2.9g

Spicy Almonds

Prep Time: 10 minutes
Cook Time: 30 minutes
Servings: 12
Ingredients:
• 1 tablespoon stevia
• 1½ teaspoons kosher salt
• 1 teaspoon paprika
• ½ teaspoon ground cinnamon
• ½ teaspoon ground cumin
• ¼ teaspoon cayenne pepper
• 1 large egg white, room temperature
• 2½ cups unblanched almonds
Preparation:
1. Preheat the oven to 325°F. Combine the first 6 ingredients in a small bowl.
2. Whisk the egg white in a separate small dish until it becomes frothy. Add the almonds and spice mixture and toss to coat.
3. Spread the mixture in a single layer in a greased baking dish. Bake in the preheated oven for 30 minutes, stirring every 10 minutes.

4. Allow the cooked almonds to cool completely on waxed paper. Store in an airtight container.
5. Serve and enjoy!
Serving Suggestion: Serve with tea.
Variation Tip: You can also add ground coriander.
Nutritional Information per Serving:
Calories: 230|Fat: 20g|Sat Fat: 2g|Carbohydrates: 9g|Fiber: 4g|Sugar: 3g|Protein: 8g

Fish Tacos

Prep Time: 10 minutes
Cook Time: 20 minutes
Servings: 6
Ingredients:
- ¼ cup olive oil
- 1 teaspoon ground cardamom
- 1 teaspoon paprika
- 1 teaspoon salt
- 1 teaspoon pepper
- 6 mahi-mahi fillets
- 12 corn tortillas
- 2 cups red cabbage, chopped
- 1 cup fresh cilantro, chopped
- 2 medium limes, cut into wedges
- Hot pepper sauce
Preparation:
1. Combine the first five ingredients in a baking dish. Add the fillets and toss to coat. Refrigerate for 30 minutes, covered.
2. Drain the fish and toss out the marinade. Grill the fillets, covered, in a greased grill pan over medium-high heat until the flesh flakes easily with a fork, about 4–5 minutes on each side.
3. Remove the fish from the pan. Heat the tortillas for 30–45 seconds on the grill pan.
4. To assemble the tacos, divide the fish among the tortillas and top with the red cabbage and cilantro.
5. Fold the sides of the tortilla over the fish mixture and squeeze a little lime juice and spicy pepper sauce over the top.
6. Serve and enjoy!
Serving Suggestion: Serve with lime wedges.
Variation Tip: You can also add salsa verde.
Nutritional Information per Serving:
Calories: 284|Fat: 5g|Sat Fat: 1g|Carbohydrates: 26g|Fiber: 4g|Sugar: 2g|Protein: 35g

Warm Rice and Pintos

Prep Time: 15 minutes
Cook Time: 15 minutes
Servings: 4
Ingredients:
- 1 tablespoon olive oil
- 1 cup frozen corn
- 1 small onion, chopped
- 2 garlic cloves, minced
- 1½ teaspoons chili powder
- 1½ teaspoons ground cumin
- 1 can pinto beans, rinsed and drained
- 1 package ready-to-serve brown rice
- 1 can chopped green chiles
- ½ cup salsa
- ¼ cup fresh cilantro, chopped
- 1 bunch romaine, quartered lengthwise through the core
Preparation:
1. Heat the oil in a large skillet. Stir in the corn and onion and cook for 4–5 minutes, or until the onion is soft.
2. Cook for another minute after adding the garlic, chili powder, and cumin.
3. Add and heat through, stirring occasionally, the beans, rice, green chiles, salsa, and cilantro.
4. Serve with romaine wedges on the side.
5. Serve and enjoy!
Serving Suggestion: Serve with any sauce.
Variation Tip: You can sprinkle with cheese.
Nutritional Information per Serving:
Calories: 331|Fat: 8g|Sat Fat: 2g|Carbohydrates: 50g|Fiber: 9g|Sugar: 5g|Protein: 12g

Cilantro Lime Shrimp

Prep Time: 10 minutes
Cook Time: 20 minutes
Servings: 4
Ingredients:
- $1/3$ cup fresh cilantro, chopped
- 1½ teaspoons lime zest, grated
- $1/3$ cup lime juice
- 1 jalapeno pepper, seeded and minced
- 2 tablespoons olive oil
- 3 garlic cloves, minced
- ¼ teaspoon salt
- ¼ teaspoon ground cumin
- ¼ teaspoon pepper
- 1 pound uncooked shrimp, peeled and deveined
- Lime slices

Preparation:
1. Toss the shrimp with the first nine ingredients. Allow 15 minutes for cooling.
2. Thread 4 metal or water-soaked wooden skewers with the marinaded shrimp and lime slices. Cover and grill over medium heat for 2–4 minutes per side, or until the shrimp turn pink.
3. Serve and enjoy!
Serving Suggestion: Serve with garlic sauce.
Variation Tip: Sprinkle cilantro on top.
Nutritional Information per Serving:
Calories: 167|Fat: 8g|Sat Fat: 1g|Carbohydrates: 4g|Fiber: 0g|Sugar: 1g|Protein: 19g

Sweet Potatoes

Prep Time: 10 minutes
Cook Time: 45 minutes
Servings: 4
Ingredients:
- 4 medium sweet potatoes
- ½ cup fat-free coconut Greek yogurt
- 1 medium apple, chopped
- ¼ cup unsweetened coconut flakes, toasted

Preparation:
1. Preheat the oven to 400°F. Place the potatoes on a baking sheet lined with foil. Bake for 45–60 minutes, or until they soften.
2. Cut an "X" in each potato using a sharp knife. Using a fork, fluff the pulp. Add the remaining ingredients on top.
3. Serve and enjoy!
Serving Suggestion: Top with maple syrup.
Variation Tip: You can skip apple.
Nutritional Information per Serving:
Calories: 321|Fat: 3g|Sat Fat: 2g|Carbohydrates: 70g|Fiber: 8g|Sugar: 30g|Protein: 7g

Strawberries and Cream Cheese Crepes

Prep Time: 10 minutes
Cook Time: 10 minutes
Serves: 4
Ingredients
- 4 tbsp. cream cheese, softened
- 2 tbsp. sifted powdered sugar
- 2 tsp. vanilla extract
- 2 prepackaged crepes, each about 8 inches in diameter
- 8 strawberries, hulled and sliced
- 1 tsp. powdered sugar for garnish
- 2 tbsp. caramel sauce, warmed

Preparation
1. Heat the oven to 325°F. Lightly coat a baking dish with cooking spray.
2. In a mixing bowl, blend the cream cheese until smooth using an electric mixer. Add the powdered sugar and vanilla. Mix well.
3. Spread ½ of the cream cheese mixture on each crepe, leaving ½-inch around the edge. Top with 2 tbsp. of strawberries.
4. Roll up each crepe and place seam-side down in the prepared baking dish. Bake until lightly browned (about 10 minutes).
5. Cut the crepes in half. Transfer to four individual serving plates.

Serving Suggestion: Sprinkle each crepe with powdered sugar and top with ½ tbsp. of caramel sauce. Serve immediately.

Variation Tip: Using whipped cream cheese in these crepes instead of regular cream cheese saves one-third of the calories, fat, and sodium. The recipe works with other berries as well as stone fruit such as sliced peaches or apricots.

Nutritional Information Per Serving:
Calories 143 | Protein 3g | Carbohydrate 17g | Dietary fiber 0.5g | Fat 7g | Sugars 7g | Sodium 161mg

Apple-Berry Cobbler

Prep Time: 55 minutes
Cook Time: 40 minutes
Serves: 6
Ingredients
The Filling:
- 1 cup fresh raspberries
- 1 cup fresh blueberries
- 2 cups chopped apples
- 2 tbsp. turbinado or brown sugar
- ½ tsp. ground cinnamon
- 1 tsp. lemon zest
- 2 tsp. lemon juice
- 1½ tbsp. cornstarch

The Topping:
- Egg white from 1 large egg
- ¼ cup soy milk
- ¼ tsp. salt
- ½ tsp. vanilla
- 1½ tbsp. turbinado or brown sugar
- ¾ cup whole-wheat pastry flour

Preparation
1. Heat the oven to 350°F. Lightly coat six individual ovenproof ramekins with cooking spray.
2. Add the raspberries, blueberries, apples, sugar, cinnamon, lemon zest, and lemon juice in a medium bowl. Stir to mix evenly.
3. Add the cornstarch and stir until it dissolves. Set aside.
4. In a separate bowl, add the egg white and whisk until lightly beaten. Add the soy milk, salt, vanilla, sugar, and pastry flour. Stir to mix well.
5. Divide the fruit mixture evenly among the prepared ramekins. Pour the topping over each. Arrange the ramekins on a large baking pan and place them in the oven.
6. Bake until the filling is tender and the topping is golden brown (about 30 minutes).

Serving Suggestion: Serve warm.

Variation Tip: Add more berries if desired.

Nutritional Information Per Serving:
Calories 119 | Protein 3.5g | Carbohydrate24 g | Dietary fiber 4g | Sugars 12 g | Fat 0g | Sodium 114mg

133

Vanilla Poached Peaches

Prep Time: 10 minutes
Cook Time: 30 minutes
Serves: 4
Ingredients
- 1 cup water
- ½ cup sugar
- 1 vanilla bean, split and scraped
- 4 large peaches, pitted and quartered
- Mint leaves or ground cinnamon, for garnish

Preparation
1. Place the water, sugar, vanilla bean (and scrapings) into a saucepan. Over low heat, stir the mixture until the sugar dissolves. Continue to simmer until the mixture thickens (about 10 minutes).
2. Add the cut fruit. Poach over low heat for about 5 minutes.

Serving Suggestion: Transfer the peaches and sauce to small, decorative bowls. Garnish with mint leaves or a dusting of cinnamon. Serve immediately.

Variation Tip: You can substitute 4 nectarines, 4 apples, 4 small pears, or 8 apricots in place of the peaches.

Nutritional Information Per Serving:
Calories 156 | Protein 1g | Carbohydrate 38g | Dietary fiber 2g | Sugars 24g | Fat 0.1g | Sodium 2mg

Mixed Berry Whole-Grain Cake

Prep Time: 15 minutes
Cook Time: 35 minutes
Serves: 8
Ingredients
- ½ cup skim milk
- 1 tbsp. vinegar
- 2 tbsp. canola oil
- 1 tsp. vanilla
- 1 egg
- ⅓ cup packed brown sugar
- 1 cup whole-wheat pastry flour
- ½ tsp. baking soda
- ½ tsp. ground cinnamon
- ⅛ tsp. salt
- 1 cup frozen mixed berries, such as blueberries, raspberries, and blackberries (do not thaw)
- ¼ cup low-fat granola, slightly crushed

Preparation
1. Heat the oven to 350°F. Spray an 8-inch round cake pan with cooking spray and coat with flour.
2. In a large bowl, mix the milk, vinegar, oil, vanilla, egg, and brown sugar until smooth.
3. Stir in the flour, baking soda, cinnamon, and salt just until moistened.
4. Gently fold half the berries into the batter.
5. Spoon the mixture into the prepared pan. Sprinkle with the remaining berries and top with the granola.
6. Bake for 25 to 30 minutes or until golden brown and the top springs back when touched in the center.
7. Cool in the pan on a cooling rack for 10 minutes.

Serving Suggestion: Serve with low-fat ice cream.
Variation Tip: Fresh berries work as well as frozen ones in this delicious year-round treat.
Nutritional Information Per Serving:
Calories 165 | Protein 4g | Carbohydrate 26g | Dietary fiber 3g | Sugars 9g | Fat 5g | Sodium 153mg

Ambrosia With Coconut and Toasted Almonds

Prep Time: 15 minutes
Cook Time: 30 minutes
Serves: 8
Ingredients
- ½ cup slivered almonds
- ½ cup unsweetened shredded coconut
- 1 small pineapple, cubed (about 3 cups)
- 5 oranges, segmented
- 2 red apples, cored and diced
- 1 banana, halved lengthwise, peeled, and sliced crosswise
- 2 tbsp. cream sherry
- Fresh mint leaves for garnish

Preparation
1. Heat the oven to 325°F. Spread the almonds on a baking sheet and bake, stirring occasionally, until golden and fragrant for about 10 minutes. Transfer immediately to a plate to cool.
2. Add the coconut to the sheet and bake, stirring often, until lightly browned for about 10 minutes. Transfer immediately to a plate to cool.

3. In a large bowl, combine the pineapple, oranges, apples, banana, and sherry. Toss gently to mix well.
Serving Suggestion: Divide the fruit mixture evenly among individual bowls. Sprinkle evenly with the toasted almonds and coconut and garnish with the mint.
Variation Tip: Add honey according to your taste.
Nutritional Information Per Serving:
Calories 177 | Protein 3g | Carbohydrate 30g | Dietary fiber 6g | Sugars 0g | Fat 5g | Sodium 2mg

Almond and Apricot Biscotti

Prep Time: 15 minutes
Cook Time: 45 minutes
Serves: 24
Ingredients
- ¾ cup whole-wheat (whole-meal) flour
- ¾ cup all-purpose (plain) flour
- ¼ cup firmly packed brown sugar
- 1 tsp. baking powder
- 2 eggs, lightly beaten
- 2 tbsp. 1 percent low-fat milk
- 2 tbsp. canola oil
- 2 tbsp. dark honey
- ½ tsp. almond extract
- ²/₃ cup chopped dried apricots
- ¼ cup coarsely chopped almonds

Preparation
1. Heat the oven to 350°F.
2. In a large bowl, combine the flours, brown sugar, and baking powder. Whisk to blend.
3. Add the eggs, milk, canola oil, honey, and almond extract. Stir with a wooden spoon until the dough just begins to come together.
4. Add the chopped apricots and almonds. With floured hands, mix until the dough is well-blended.
5. Place the dough on a long sheet of plastic wrap and shape by hand into a flattened log 12 inches long, 3 inches wide, and about 1 inch high. Lift the plastic wrap to invert the dough onto a non-stick baking sheet.
6. Bake until lightly browned (25 to 30 minutes). Transfer to another baking sheet to cool for 10 minutes. Leave the oven set at 350°F.
7. Place the cooled log on a cutting board. With a serrated knife, cut crosswise on the diagonal into 24 slices, ½-inch wide. Arrange the slices, cut-side down, on the baking sheet. Return to the oven and bake until crisp for 15 to 20 minutes.

8. Transfer to a wire rack and let cool completely. Store in an airtight container.
Serving Suggestion: Serve with tea.
Variation Tip: Add more sweetener according to taste.
Nutritional Information Per Serving:
Calories 75 | Protein 2g | Carbohydrate 12g | Dietary fiber 1g | Sugars 2g | Fat 2g | Sodium 17mg

Baked Apples with Cherries and Almonds

Prep Time: 20 minutes
Cook Time: 60 minutes
Serves: 6
Ingredients
- ¹/₃ cup dried cherries, coarsely chopped
- 3 tbsp. chopped almonds
- 1 tbsp. wheat germ
- 1 tbsp. firmly packed brown sugar
- ½ tsp. ground cinnamon
- ¹/₈ tsp. ground nutmeg
- 6 small Golden Delicious apples, about 1¾ lbs. total weight
- ½ cup apple juice
- ¼ cup water
- 2 tbsp. dark honey
- 2 tsp. walnut oil or canola oil

Preparation
1. Preheat the oven to 350°F.
2. In a small bowl, toss together the cherries, almonds, wheat germ, brown sugar, cinnamon, and nutmeg until all the ingredients are evenly mixed. Set aside.
3. The apples can be left unpeeled if you like. To peel the apples decoratively, with a vegetable peeler or a sharp knife, remove the peel from each apple in a circular motion, skipping every other row so that rows of peel alternate with rows of apple flesh. Working from the stem end, core each apple, stopping ¾-inch from the bottom.
4. Divide the cherry mixture evenly among the apples, pressing the mixture gently into each cavity.
5. Arrange the apples upright in a heavy ovenproof frying pan or small baking dish just large enough to hold them. Pour the apple juice and water into the pan. Drizzle the honey and oil evenly over the apples, and cover the pan snugly with aluminum foil.
6. Bake until the apples are tender when pierced with a knife (50 to 60 minutes).
Serving Suggestion: Transfer the apples to individual plates and drizzle with the pan juices. Serve warm or at room temperature.
Variation Tip: Add nuts of your choice.
Nutritional Information Per Serving:
Calories 200 | Protein 2g | Carbohydrate 39g | Dietary fiber 5g | Sugars 8g | Fat 4g | Sodium 7mg

Rainbow Ice Pops

Prep Time: 5 minutes
Cook Time: 1 hour
Serves: 6
Ingredients
- ½ cups diced strawberries, cantaloupe, and watermelon
- ½ cup blueberries
- 2 cups 100% apple juice
- 6 paper cups (6–8 oz. each)
- 6 craft sticks

Preparation
1. Mix the fruit together and divide it evenly into the paper cups. Pour ⅓ cup of the apple juice into each paper cup.
2. Place the cups on a level surface in the freezer. Freeze until partially frozen (approximately 1 hour). Insert a stick into the center of each cup. Freeze until firm.

Serving Suggestion: Serve cooled.
Variation Tip: Add some sweetener according to your taste.
Nutritional Information Per Serving:
Calories 60 | Protein 0.5g | Carbohydrate 14g | Dietary fiber 1g | Sugars 0g | Fat 0.1g | Sodium 6mg

Lemon Pudding Cakes

Prep Time: 15 minutes
Cook Time: 40 minutes
Serves: 2
Ingredients:
- 2 eggs
- ¼ teaspoon salt
- ¾ cup sugar
- 1 cup skim milk
- ⅓ cup freshly squeezed lemon juice
- 3 tablespoons all-purpose flour
- 1 tablespoon finely grated lemon peel
- 1 tablespoon melted butter

Preparation:
1. Preheat the oven to 350°F.
2. Grease two custard cups with cooking oil.
3. Whisk the egg whites with ¼ cup of sugar in a mixer until the mixture forms stiff peaks.
4. Beat the egg yolks with ½ cup of sugar until mixed.
5. Stir in the lemon juice, milk, butter, flour, and lemon peel. Mix until smooth.
6. Fold in the egg white mixture to the yolk mixture.
7. Divide the batter into the custard cups.
8. Bake them for 40 minutes until golden on top.
9. Serve.

Serving Suggestion: Serve with a scoop of ice cream on the side.
Variation Tip: Add lemon curd on top.
Nutritional Information per Serving:
Calories 182 | Fat 6g |Sodium 20mg | Carbs 15g | Fiber 2g | Sugar 1.2g | Protein 1.2g

Rustic Apple-Cranberry Tart

Prep Time: 1 hour
Cook Time: 90 minutes
Serves: 8
Ingredients
The Filling:
- ½ cup dried cranberries
- ¼ cup apple juice
- 2 tbsp. cornstarch
- 4 large tart apples, cored, peeled, and sliced
- 1 tsp. vanilla extract
- ¼ tsp. ground cinnamon

The Crust:
- 1¼ cups whole-wheat (whole-meal) flour
- 2 tsp. sugar
- 3 tbsp. trans-free margarine
- ¼ cup ice water

Preparation
1. In a small microwave-safe bowl, combine the cranberries and apple juice. Cook on high for 1 minute, then stir. Continue to heat for 30 seconds at a time, stirring after each interval, until the apple juice is very hot. Cover and set aside until the mixture is close to room temperature (about 1 hour).
2. Heat the oven to 375°F.

3. In a large bowl, combine the cornstarch and apple slices. Toss well to coat evenly.

4. Add the cranberries and juice. Mix well. Stir in the vanilla and cinnamon. Set aside.

5. To prepare the crust, add the flour and sugar to a large mixing bowl. Using a fork or pastry cutter, cut in the margarine until the mixture is crumbly. Add the ice water 1 tbsp. at a time and mix with a fork until the dough begins to form a rough mass.

6. Tape a large piece of aluminum foil onto the countertop. Sprinkle it with flour. Place the dough in the center of the foil and flatten.

7. Roll the dough from the center to the edges using a rolling pin, making a circle of about 13 inches in diameter.

8. Place the fruit filling in the center of the dough. Spread the filling over the dough, leaving a 1 to 2-inch border. Fold the edges of the crust up and over the filling. The pastry won't cover all of the filling (it should look rustic).

9. Remove the tape from the foil and countertop. Place another piece of foil over the tart to protect the exposed fruit. Slide the tart (bottom and top foil included) onto a cookie sheet and bake for about 30 minutes.

10. Remove the top foil and continue baking until browned (about 10 minutes).

Serving Tip: Cut into eight wedges and serve immediately.

Variation Tip: Serve with a scoop of fat-free frozen yogurt or a dollop of light or fat-free whipped topping.

Nutritional Information Per Serving:
Calories 197 | Protein 3g | Carbohydrate 35g | Dietary fiber 5g | Sugar 1g | Fat 5g | Sodium 40mg

Sweet Potato and Squash Pie

Prep Time: 10 minutes
Cook Time: 1 hour
Serves: 8
Ingredients
• 1 sweet potato (about ¼ lb.), peeled and cooked
• 1 buttercup squash (about 2½ lbs.), peeled, seeded, and cooked
• ½ cup silken tofu
• ½ cup soy milk
• ¼ cup egg whites
• ¼ cup rye flour
• ½ tsp. each clove, cinnamon, nutmeg, and vanilla extract
• 1 tsp. freshly grated ginger
• 1 tsp. orange zest
• 3 tbsp. honey
• 1 frozen pre-made 9-inch pie shell

Preparation
1. Heat the oven to 300°F.
2. Puree the sweet potato and squash in a food processor. Place in a large bowl.
3. Add the remaining ingredients and mix together until smooth and well-combined.
4. Place the pie shell on a sheet pan. Pour the mixture into the pie shell and bake for 45 to 55 minutes or until the internal temperature is 180°F.

Serving Suggestion: Serve with tea.
Variation Tip: Add sweetener according to your taste.
Nutritional Information Per Serving:
Calories 210 | Protein 5g | Carbohydrate 34g | Dietary fiber 4g | Sugars 7g | Fat 6g | Sodium 109mg

Yogurt Cheesecake

Prep Time: 10 minutes
Cook Time: 35 minutes
Serves: 4
Ingredients:
• 1¼ cups fat-free Greek yogurt
• 2 tablespoons arrowroot starch
• 1½ egg whites
• ½ cup cocoa powder
• ½ teaspoon organic vanilla extract

Preparation:
1. Preheat the baking oven to 350° F and grease a cake pan.
2. Meanwhile, add everything in a bowl and mix well.
3. Pour the mixture in the cake pan and bake for about 35 minutes.
4. Take out and set aside to cool.
5. Refrigerate for three to four hours, slice and serve.

Serving Suggestions: Top with strawberry syrup before serving.
Variation Tip: You can also add stevia to enhance taste.
Nutritional Information per Serving:
Calories: 180 | Fat: 5.6g | Sat Fat: 3.3g | Carbohydrates: 26.8g | Fiber: 3.3g | Sugar: 16.4g | Protein: 11.7g

Peaches a la Mode

Prep Time: 20 minutes
Cook Time: 30 minutes
Serves: 2
Ingredients
- 2 medium peaches, peeled and thinly sliced
- $1/8$ tsp. cinnamon
- $1/3$ cup low-fat granola
- 1 cup fat-free vanilla ice cream

Preparation
1. Heat the oven to 350°F. Lightly coat a small baking dish with cooking spray.
2. Place the peaches in the baking dish. Sprinkle with the cinnamon and granola. Bake until the fruit is bubbling (about 30 minutes).
3. Let cool for 5 to 10 minutes.

Serving Suggestion: Divide the ice cream into two bowls (½ cup each). Top each with half of the baked peaches. Serve immediately.
Variation Tip: For a variation of this classic dessert, try berries, apples, pears, plums, or nectarines instead of peaches. Or, if you prefer, try a combination of any of these fruits.
Nutritional Information Per Serving:
Calories 221 | Protein 5g | Carbohydrate 48g | Dietary fiber 4g | Sugars 9g | Fat 5g | Sodium 105mg

Mixed Berry Coffee Cake

Prep Time: 15 minutes
Cook Time: 30 minutes
Serves: 6
Ingredients:
- ½ cup skim milk
- 1 tablespoon vinegar
- 2 tablespoons canola oil
- 1 teaspoon vanilla
- 1 egg
- $1/3$ cup packed brown sugar
- 1 cup whole-wheat pastry flour
- ½ teaspoon baking soda
- ½ teaspoon ground cinnamon
- $1/8$ teaspoon salt
- 1 cup frozen mixed berries
- ¼ cup low-fat granola, crushed

Preparation:
1. Preheat the oven to 350°F.
2. Grease an 8-inch baking pan with cooking spray and then dust it with flour.
3. Combine the milk with the vanilla, oil, vinegar, brown sugar, and egg until smooth.
4. Add the baking soda, cinnamon, salt, and flour. Mix well.
5. Fold in half of the berries and transfer the batter to the pan.
6. Top it with the remaining berries and the granola.
7. Bake for 30 minutes until golden brown.
8. Serve.

Serving Suggestion: Serve with chocolate sauce on top.
Variation Tip: Add chocolate chips or sprinkles on top.
Nutritional Information per Serving:
Calories 135 | Fat 23g |Sodium 50mg | Carbs 22g | Fiber 3g | Sugar 4g | Protein 4g

Fruit Cake

Prep Time: 20 minutes
Cook Time: 30 minutes
Serves: 12
Ingredients
- 2 cups assorted chopped dried fruit, such as cherries, currants, dates, or figs
- ½ cup unsweetened applesauce
- ½ cup crushed pineapple packed in juice, drained
- Zest and juice of 1 medium orange
- Zest and juice of 1 lemon
- ½ cup unsweetened apple juice
- 2 tbsp. real vanilla extract
- ¼ cup sugar
- ½ cup rolled oats
- ¼ cup flaxseed flour
- 1 cup whole-wheat pastry flour
- ½ tsp. baking soda
- ½ tsp. baking powder
- 1 egg
- ½ cup crushed or chopped walnuts

Preparation
1. Preheat the oven to 325°F.
2. Combine the dried fruit, applesauce, pineapple, fruit zests and juices, and vanilla in a medium bowl. Let the mixture soak for 15 to 20 minutes.
3. Line the bottom of a 9 x 4-inch pan with parchment paper.
4. Whisk together the sugar, oats, flours, baking soda, and baking powder in a large bowl.

5. Add the fruit and liquid mixture to the dry ingredients and stir to combine.
6. Add the egg and walnuts and stir to combine.
7. Pour the mixture into the loaf pan and bake for 1 hour, or until a toothpick inserted in the center comes out clean.
8. Let the fruitcake cool for 30 minutes before removing it from the pan.
Serving Suggestions: Serve with tea.
Variation Tip: Add nuts of your choice.
Nutritional Information Per Serving:
Calories 229 | Protein 5g | Carbohydrate 41g | Dietary fiber 5g | Sugar 5g | Fat 3g | Sodium 117mg

Carrot Cake Cookies

Prep Time: 10 minutes
Cook Time: 15 minutes
Serves: 6
Ingredients:
• ½ cup applesauce
• ½ cup brown sugar
• ½ cup sugar
• ½ cup oil
• 2 eggs
• 1 teaspoon vanilla extract
• 1 cup flour
• 1 cup whole-wheat flour
• 1 teaspoon baking soda
• 1 teaspoon baking powder
• ¼ teaspoon salt
• 1 teaspoon ground cinnamon
• ½ teaspoon ground nutmeg
• ½ teaspoon ground ginger
• 2 cups old-fashioned rolled oats
• 1½ cups finely grated carrots
• 1 cup raisins or golden raisins
Preparation:
1. Preheat the oven to 350°F.
2. Mix the applesauce with the eggs, oil, sugars, and vanilla in a bowl.
3. Stir in all the dry ingredients.
4. Mix well, then fold in the carrots and raisins.
5. Drop a tablespoon of cookie dough on a cookie sheet.
6. Add more cookies drop by drop.
7. Bake the cookies 15 minutes until golden brown.
8. Serve.
Serving Suggestion: Serve the cookies with your favorite hot beverage.

Variation Tip: Add lemon zest to the cookie dough.
Nutritional Information per Serving:
Calories 124 | Fat 5g |Sodium 32mg | Carbs 31g | Fiber 0.3g | Sugar 1g | Protein 5.7g

Warm Chocolate Pudding

Prep Time: 10 minutes
Cook Time: 10 minutes
Serves: 6
Ingredients
• 1 tbsp. ground flaxseeds (flax meal)
• 3 tbsp. brewed espresso
• 2¼ cups skim milk, divided
• ⅔ cup sugar, divided
• ⅛ tsp. salt
• ⅔ cup unsweetened cocoa powder
• 1 tsp. vanilla extract
• 2 tbsp. cornstarch
Preparation
1. Lightly beat the ground flaxseeds (flax meal) with the warm espresso with a fork in a medium bowl. Set aside.
2. In a medium saucepan, combine 1½ cups milk, ⅓ cup sugar, and salt. Bring to a simmer over medium heat, stirring occasionally.
3. Meanwhile, whisk the remaining ⅓ cup sugar, cocoa powder, and cornstarch in a medium bowl.
4. Then whisk in the remaining ¾ cup milk until blended. Whisk the simmering milk mixture into the cocoa mixture.
5. Pour the mixture back into the saucepan and bring it to a simmer over medium heat, whisking constantly, until thickened and glossy (about 3 minutes). Remove from the heat.
6. Whisk about 1 cup of the hot cocoa mixture into the beaten flaxseeds. Add this mixture to the saucepan and cook over medium-low heat, whisking constantly, until steaming and thickened (about 2 minutes). Do not let the mixture boil.
Serving Tip: Whisk in the vanilla extract. Serve warm.
Variation Tip: Add eggs instead of flaxseeds.
Nutritional Information Per Serving:
Calories 169 | Protein 5g | Carbohydrate 35g | Dietary fiber 2g | Sugar 22g | Fat 1g | Sodium 86mg

Strawberries Cream Cheese Crepes

Prep Time: 15 minutes
Cook Time: 10 minutes
Serves: 4
Ingredients:
- 4 tablespoons cream cheese, softened
- 2 tablespoons powdered sugar, sifted
- 2 teaspoons vanilla extract
- 2 tortilla wraps
- 8 strawberries, hulled and sliced

Preparation:
1. Preheat the oven to 325°F. Grease a baking dish with cooking spray.
2. Blend the cream cheese with the vanilla and powdered sugar in a mixer.
3. Spread the cream cheese mixture on each tortilla and top them with 2 tablespoons of strawberries.
4. Roll the tortillas and place them in the baking dish.
5. Bake them for 10 minutes until golden brown.
6. Garnish as desired.
7. Serve.

Serving Suggestion: Serve with strawberry sauce on top.
Variation Tip: Add other berries to the wrap as well.
Nutritional Information per Serving:
Calories 144 | Fat 4.9g |Sodium 13mg | Carbs 19.3g | Fiber 1.9g | Sugar 9.7g | Protein 3.4g

Apple Dumplings

Prep Time: 15 minutes
Cook Time: 30 minutes
Serves: 6
Ingredients:
Dough:
- 1 tablespoon butter
- 1 teaspoon honey
- 1 cup whole-wheat flour
- 2 tablespoons buckwheat flour
- 2 tablespoons rolled oats
- 2 tablespoons brandy or apple liquor

Apple filling:
- 6 large tart apples, sliced
- 1 teaspoon nutmeg
- 2 tablespoons honey
- Zest of one lemon

Preparation:
1. Combine the flours with the oats, honey, and butter in a food processor.
2. Pulse this mixture a few times, then stir in the apple liquor or brandy.
3. Mix until it forms a dough. Wrap it in plastic wrap and refrigerate it for 2 hours.
4. Preheat the oven to 350°F.
5. Mix the apples with the honey, nutmeg, and lemon zest, then set the mixture aside.
6. Take the dough out of the refrigerator and spread it into a ¼-inch thick sheet.
7. Cut it into 8-inch circles and then layer greased muffin cups with the dough circles.
8. Divide the apple mixture into the muffin cups and seal the dough at the top.
9. Bake for 30 minutes until golden brown.
10. Enjoy.

Serving Suggestion: Serve with apple sauce on the side.
Variation Tip: Add a tablespoon of Nutella to the dumplings.
Nutritional Information per Serving:
Calories 178 | Fat 3.1g |Sodium 13mg | Carbs 32g | Fiber 2.5g | Sugar 15g | Protein 6g

Berries in Balsamic Vinegar

Prep Time: 15 minutes
Cook Time: 0 minutes
Serves: 4
Ingredients:
- ¼ cup balsamic vinegar
- 2 tablespoons brown sugar
- 1 teaspoon vanilla extract
- ½ cup strawberries, sliced
- ½ cup blueberries
- ½ cup raspberries
- 2 shortbread biscuits

Preparation:

1. Combine the balsamic vinegar, vanilla, and brown sugar in a small bowl.
2. Toss the strawberries with raspberries and blueberries in a bowl.
3. Pour the vinegar mixture on top and marinate them for 15 minutes.
4. Add the biscuits to a serving bowl.
5. Spread the marinated berries on top of the biscuits.
6. Serve immediately.

Serving Suggestion: Serve with a scoop of ice cream on the side.

Variation Tip: Add a sprinkling of crushed candy on top.

Nutritional Information per Serving:
Calories 110 | Fat 1.2g |Sodium 70mg | Carbs 31g | Fiber 12.4g | Sugar 4.2g | Protein 12g

Sweet Potato Pie

Prep Time: 10 minutes
Cook Time: 45 minutes
Serves: 6
Ingredients:
• 1 sweet potato, peeled and cooked
• 1 buttercup squash, peeled and cooked
• ½ cup silken tofu
• ½ cup soy milk
• ¼ cup egg whites
• ¼ cup rye flour
• ½ teaspoon each clove, cinnamon, nutmeg, and vanilla extract
• 1 teaspoon fresh ginger, grated
• 1 teaspoon orange zest
• 3 tablespoons honey
• 1 frozen pre-made 9-inch pie shell

Preparation:
1. Puree the squash with the sweet potato in a processor.
2. Transfer the mixture to a bowl and mix in the other ingredients.
3. Spread the pie shell in a baking pan and pour the pumpkin mixture into it.
4. Bake for 45 minutes.
5. Slice and serve.

Serving Suggestion: Serve with pecans on top.
Variation Tip: Add whipped cream on top of the pie.
Nutritional Information per Serving:
Calories 210 | Fat 7.1g |Sodium 34mg | Carbs 27.1g | Fiber 0.2g | Sugar 11.3g | Protein 4.6g

Walnut Chocolate Chip Cookies

Prep Time: 10 minutes
Cook Time: 15 minutes
Serves: 6
Ingredients:
• 2 cups rolled oats
• ½ cup all-purpose flour
• ½ cup whole-wheat pastry flour
• 1 teaspoon ground cinnamon
• ½ teaspoon baking soda
• ½ teaspoon salt
• ½ cup tahini
• 4 tablespoons unsalted butter, cut into pieces
• ⅔ cup granulated sugar
• ⅔ cup packed light brown sugar
• 1 large egg
• 1 large egg white
• 1 tablespoon vanilla extract
• 1 cup semisweet or bittersweet chocolate chips
• ½ cup chopped walnuts

Preparation:
1. Preheat the oven to 350°F.
2. Layer 2 baking sheets with parchment paper.
3. Mix the oats with both of the flours, baking soda, and cinnamon in a bowl.
4. Beat the butter with the tahini in an electric mixer.
5. Whisk in the sugars and beat well.
6. Stir in the eggs, egg white, and vanilla while beating continuously.
7. Add the oats mixture and mix well.
8. Fold in the walnuts and chocolate chips.
9. Prepare cookie balls out of this dough and place them on the baking sheets.
10. Lightly press each ball using your finger.
11. Bake for 16 minutes until golden brown.
12. Allow them to cool for 2 minutes.
13. Serve.

Serving Suggestion: Serve with chocolate sauce on the side.
Variation Tip: Add shredded coconut to the cookies.
Nutritional Information per Serving:
Calories 221 | Fat 5.7g |Sodium 47mg | Carbs 12.4g | Fiber 1.2g | Sugar 15g | Protein 10.3g

Chocolate Pudding

Prep Time: 10 minutes
Cook Time: 5 minutes
Serves: 2
Ingredients:
- 3 tablespoons cornstarch
- 2 tablespoons cocoa powder
- 2 tablespoons sugar
- ⅛ teaspoon salt
- 2 cups non-fat milk
- ⅓ cup chocolate chips
- ½ teaspoon vanilla extract

Preparation:
1. Mix the cornstarch with the sugar and cocoa powder in a saucepan.
2. Stir in the milk and cook on medium heat until the mixture thickens.
3. Turn off the heat, then fold in the chocolate chips and vanilla.
4. Mix until well combined.
5. Divide the pudding into serving glasses and allow them to chill.
6. Serve.

Serving Suggestion: Serve with whipped cream on top.
Variation Tip: Add raspberries on top of the puddings.
Nutritional Information per Serving:
Calories 318 | Fat 1.7g |Sodium 79mg | Carbs 28.8g | Fiber 0.1g | Sugar 0.3g | Protein 4.9g

Dark Chocolate Kefir Parfait

Prep Time: 15 minutes
Cook Time: 0 minutes
Serves: 1
Ingredients:
- ⅔ cup plain low-fat kefir
- 1 tablespoon mini dark chocolate chips
- 1 tablespoon shredded unsweetened coconut
- ½ cup frozen unsweetened yogurt, softened

Preparation:
1. Add the kefir to a large serving glass.
2. Top it with the frozen yogurt.
3. Garnish with the chocolate chips and coconut.
4. Serve.

Serving Suggestion: Serve the parfait with sweet pound cake slices.
Variation Tip: Add a sprinkle of almond flakes on top.
Nutritional Information per Serving:
Calories 178 | Fat 19g |Sodium 14mg | Carbs 13g | Fiber 0.3g | Sugar 1g | Protein 3g

Strawberry Trifle

Prep Time: 10 minutes
Cook Time: 0 minutes
Serves: 4
Ingredients:
- 2 pears, pared, cored, and thinly sliced
- 2 tablespoons lemon juice
- 2 cups strawberries, chopped
- ½ teaspoon almond extract
- 2 tablespoons orange juice
- 2 tablespoons honey
- ½ of 9-inch angel food cake, cut into 1-inch cubes
- 3 cups vanilla yogurt

Preparation:
1. Mix the pears with the lemon juice, almond extract, and strawberries in a bowl.
2. Whisk the honey with the orange juice in another bowl.
3. Layer each serving glass: with ⅓ full of cake cubes, 1 tablespoon orange juice mixture, 1 cup yogurt, 1 cup pear, and 1 cup strawberries.
4. Top each glass with the remaining yogurt.
5. Refrigerate for 1 to 2 hours.
6. Garnish with strawberries.
7. Serve.

Serving Suggestion: Serve the trifle with berry compote on top.
Variation Tip: Add whipped cream on top of the trifles.
Nutritional Information per Serving:
Calories 291 | Fat 10.2g |Sodium 76mg | Carbs 27g | Fiber 2.9g | Sugar 21.4g | Protein 8.8g

Cashew Cream Mousse

Prep Time: 50 minutes
Cook Time: 0 minutes
Serves: 2
Ingredients:
• ½ cup cashews, presoaked
• 1 tablespoon honey
• 1 teaspoon vanilla extract
• 1 large banana, sliced (reserve 4 slices for garnish)
• 1 cup plain non-fat Greek yogurt
Preparation:
1. Place the cashews in a small bowl and cover with 1 cup of water.
2. Soak at room temperature for 2 to 3 hours. Drain, rinse and set aside.
3. Place honey, vanilla extract, cashews and bananas in a blender or food processor. Blend until smooth. Place mixture in a medium bowl.
4. Fold in yogurt, mix well. Cover. Chill in the refrigerator, covered, for at least 45 minutes.
5. Portion mousse into two serving bowls.
6. Enjoy.
Serving Suggestion: Garnish each with two banana slices.
Variation Tip: Substitute honey with a sweetener of your choice.
Nutritional Information per Serving:
Calories 329 | Fat 14 g | Sodium 64 mg | Carbs 37 g | Fiber 3 g | Sugar 24 g | Protein 17 g

Cinnamon Applesauce

Prep Time: 10 minutes
Cook Time: 25 minutes
Serves: 4
Ingredients:
• 5 large apples, peeled
• ¼ cup water
• 1 cinnamon stick
• 3 cloves
• Zest of ½ lemon
• ½ teaspoon ground ginger
Preparation:
1. Cut the peeled apples into wedges, and discard the cores.
2. Place the apples, water and spices in a large pot.
3. Cover, and simmer over low heat for about 20 minutes, or until the apples are fluffy to the touch.
4. Remove the cinnamon stick and cloves, and mash the apples with a potato masher or fork to the desired consistency.
5. For super smooth applesauce, transfer the mixture to a blender, and blend in small batches.
Serving Suggestion: Serve with a sprinkle of cinnamon.
Variation Tip: Top vanilla ice cream with warm applesauce and crumbled pecans or walnuts or enjoy as is.
Nutritional Information per Serving:
Calories 157 | Fat 0.4 g | Sodium 5 mg | Carbs 41 g | Fiber 7 g | Sugar 27 g | Protein 0.4 g

Mango Rice Pudding

Prep Time: 10 minutes
Cook Time: 35 minutes
Serves: 4
Ingredients:
• 2 cups water
• ¼ teaspoon Iodized salt
• 1 cup long-grain uncooked brown rice
• 2 mediums ripe, peeled, cored mango
• 1 cup vanilla soymilk
• 1 tablespoon sugar
• ½ teaspoon ground cinnamon
• 1 teaspoon vanilla extract
Preparation:
1. Bring saltwater to a boil in a saucepan to cook rice; after a few minutes, simmer covered within 30–35 minutes until the rice absorbs the water.
2. Mash the mango with a mortar and pestle or a fork.
3. Pour milk, sugar, cinnamon and the mashed mango into the rice; cook uncovered on low heat, stirring frequently.
4. Remove the mango rice pudding from the heat, then stir in the vanilla soymilk.
5. Serve immediately.
Serving Suggestion: Top with mango slices and blueberries.
Variation Tip: Substitute soy milk with coconut milk.
Nutritional Information per Serving:
Calories 275 | Fat 3 g | Sodium 176 mg | Carbs 58 mg | Fiber 3 g | Sugar 20 g | Protein 4g

Mocha Chocolate Mousse

Prep Time: 5 minutes
Cook Time: 0 minutes
Serves: 4
Ingredients:
- 1 package (12 ounces) sugar-free chocolate chips
- Sweetener of your choice
- 1 cup boiling black coffee
- 3 eggs
- 1 teaspoon vanilla

Preparation:
1. Combine the chocolate chips and sugar in the blender.
2. Blend on high and slowly pour in the boiling coffee.
3. Keep the blender running and add the eggs, 1 at a time.
4. Turn the blender to low, add the vanilla and blend another 10 seconds.
5. Pour the mixture into glasses and set them in the freezer.
6. You can eat this frozen or just leave it in the freezer until it sets.
Serving Suggestion: Serve chilled with berries of your choice and mint leaves.
Variation Tip: Feel free to use a no-calorie sweetener of your choice.
Nutritional Information per Serving:
Calories 374 | Fat 24.6g | Sodium 202mg | Carbs 30g | Fiber 0g | Sugar 0.4g | Protein 8g

Delicious Fudge

Prep Time: 10 minutes
Cook Time: 30 minutes
Serves: 22 squares
Ingredients:
- ½ cup low-fat butter
- 12 ounces dark chocolate, chopped
- 1 teaspoon vanilla extract

- 2 cups coconut sugar
- 1 cup non-fat milk

Preparation:
1. Heat a pan with the milk over medium heat, add the sugar and the butter, stir and cook everything for 7 minutes.
2. Take this off heat, add the chocolate and whisk everything.
3. Pour this into a lined square pan, spread well, keep in the fridge for 30 minutes or more, cut into small squares, and serve.
4. Enjoy!
Serving Suggestion: Garnish with mint leaves.
Variation Tip: Substitute coconut sugar with a sweetener of your choice.
Nutritional Information per Serving:
Calories 150 | Fat 2g | Sodium 48mg | Carbs 28g | Fiber1g | Sugar 20g | Protein 6g

Mixed Fruit Bowl

Prep Time: 10 minutes
Serves: 3
Ingredients:

- ½ banana, peeled and sliced
- 1 tablespoon maple syrup
- ¼ cup fresh blueberries
- 1 tablespoon chopped almonds
- ¼ cup fresh strawberries, sliced
- ½ tablespoon fresh lemon juice
- ¼ cup cherries, pitted and chopped

Preparation:
1. Add everything in a large bowl and toss to coat well.
2. Add the mixture in serving bowls and top with chopped almonds.
3. Serve and enjoy!
Serving Suggestions: Top with chopped cashews before serving.
Variation Tip: Maple syrup can be replaced with applesauce.
Nutritional Information per Serving:
Calories: 65 | Fat: 1.2g | Sat Fat: 0.1g | Carbohydrates: 13.8g | Fiber: 1.3g | Sugar: 8.3g | Protein: 0.8g

Lime Cherry Cream

Prep Time: 10 minutes
Cook Time: 15 minutes
Serves: 4
Ingredients:
- 4 frozen bananas, peeled
- 1 cup frozen dark sweet cherries
- Zest and juice from 1 lime
- ½ teaspoon vanilla extract
- ¼ teaspoon Kosher or Sea salt

Preparation:
1. Blend the ingredients in a food processor and enjoy a frozen treat.
2. Place the bananas, cherries, lime juice, vanilla extract, and salt in a food processor.
3. Pulse until smooth, scraping the sides as needed.
4. Transfer the cream to bowls and serve.
Serving Suggestion: Top with the lime zest.
Variation Tip: Feel free to omit salt.
Nutritional Information per Serving:
Calories 150 | Fat 0 g | Sodium 147 mg | Carbs 37 g | Fiber 4 g | Sugar 21 g | Protein 2 g

Fig Bars

Prep Time: 15 minutes
Cook Time: 30 minutes
Serves: 6
Ingredients:
- 16 ounces dried figs, stemmed and chopped
- ½ cup walnuts, chopped
- ⅓ cup sugar
- ¼ cup orange juice
- 2 tablespoons hot water
- ½ cup margarine, softened
- 1 cup packed brown sugar
- 1 large egg
- 1½ cups all-purpose flour
- ½ teaspoon baking soda
- 1¼ cups old-fashioned rolled oats

Preparation:
1. Preheat the oven to 350°F. Grease a 9-inch x 13-inch baking pan.
2. Mix the figs with the sugar, walnuts, hot water, and orange juice in a bowl.

3. Beat the brown sugar with the margarine in an electric mixer until creamy.
4. Whisk in the egg and blend until smooth.
5. Stir in the baking soda and flour. Mix well.
6. Add the oats and mix well. Reserve 1 cup of the cookie dough for topping.
7. Transfer the remaining dough to the baking pan and press it gently.
8. Top the dough with the fig mixture and press it firmly into the dough.
9. Sprinkle the reserved cookie dough on top.
10. Bake for about 30 minutes.
11. Slice into small squares.
12. Serve.
Serving Suggestion: Serve the bars with a sweet cream dip.
Variation Tip: You can add raspberry preserve to the filling as well.
Nutritional Information per Serving:
Calories 266 | Fat 4.9g |Sodium 13mg | Carbs 29.3g | Fiber 2g | Sugar 3g | Protein 3.4g

Peach Parfait

Prep Time: 10 minutes
Cook Time: 5 minutes
Serves: 2
Ingredients:
- 1 cup, sliced and fresh peaches
- 1 ½ cup, low-fat or fat-free milk
- ⅛ tablespoon extract almond
- 1 cup fresh raspberry

Preparation:
1. Add milk, peaches and almond extract to the blender and allow it to smoothen up.
2. Mash the raspberries using a fork.
3. Take a glass and pour the two mixtures, raspberries and milk, into the glass.
Serving Suggestion: Garnish with mint leaves.
Variation Tip: Feel free to use almond milk.
Nutritional Information per Serving:
Calories 94 | Fat 0.4g | Sodium 95mg | Carbs 17.4g | Fiber 4.1g | Sugar 11.9g | Protein 7g

Chocolate Yogurt Pudding

Prep Time: 10 minutes
Cook Time: 10 minutes
Serves: 2
Ingredients:
- ½ cup Greek yogurt, plain, fat-free
- 1 ½ tablespoon maple syrup
- 2 tablespoons dark cocoa powder

Preparation:
1. Whisk together everything in a bowl until all the lumps have dissolved.
2. If your pudding is too thick, feel free to add a couple of teaspoons of skim milk, as each yogurt brand has its unique thickness.
3. Serve and enjoy.

Serving Suggestion: Garnish with mint leaves.
Variation Tip: Adjust the sweetness to taste by adjusting the maple syrup level to your preference.
Nutritional Information per Serving:
Calories 140 | Fat 3g | Sodium 66mg | Carbs 20g | Fiber 2g | Sugar 6g | Protein 11g

Vanilla Pumpkin Pudding

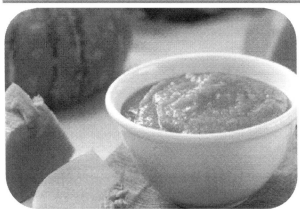

Prep Time: 10 minutes
Cook Time: 0 minutes
Serves: 6
Ingredients:
- 1½ cups fat-free vanilla yogurt
- 1 can (20 ounces) plain pumpkin purée
- ½ teaspoon ground nutmeg
- ½ teaspoon ground cinnamon
- 1 vanilla bean

Preparation:
1. Combine yogurt, pumpkin purée, nutmeg, and cinnamon in a medium-sized mixing bowl.

2. Scrape vanilla beans out of the husk and into the mixture.
3. Mix well until all ingredients are combined.
4. Chill until ready to serve.

Serving Suggestion: Top with toasted pumpkin seeds.
Variation Tip: Substitute vanilla yogurt with plain yogurt.
Nutritional Information per Serving:
Calories 95 | Fat 1.1g | Sodium 38mg | Carbs 17g | Fiber 2.1g | Sugar 3g | Protein 4.1g

Pumpkin Ice cream

Prep Time: 5 minutes
Serves: 3
Ingredients:
- 1 cup homemade pumpkin puree
- ¾ teaspoon pumpkin pie spice
- 1 cup unsweetened coconut milk
- ¼ teaspoon ground cinnamon
- ¼ cup dates, pitted and chopped
- ¼ teaspoon organic vanilla extract

Preparation:

1. Add everything in a high-speed blender and pulse until smooth.
2. Transfer the mixture in an ice cream maker and process according to manufacturer's directions.
3. Take out and transfer it in an airtight container.
4. Place it in the freezer and freeze for about three to four hours.
5. Take out, serve and enjoy!

Serving Suggestions: Top with chopped mint leaves.

Variation Tip: You can use maple syrup to enhance taste.
Nutritional Information per Serving:
Calories: 264 | Fat: 19.2g | Sat Fat: 16.9g | Carbohydrates: 23.1g | Fiber: 4.1g | Sugar: 14.1g | Protein: 3.2g

146

Dash Pear Crumble

Prep Time: 10 minutes
Cook Time: 35 minutes
Serves: 6
Ingredients:
- 5 pears, peeled, cored, and cut into large dice
- 2 tablespoons honey
- 1 tablespoon lime juice
- 2 tablespoons corn flour
- ½ teaspoon cinnamon powder
- Cooking oil spray
- 1 cup homemade granola

Preparation:
1. Place the pears, honey, lime juice, corn flour, and cinnamon in a bowl and mix well.
2. Preheat the oven to 350° F.
3. Oil an 11 by 8 ½ inch baking dish lightly, add the pear mixture, bake for 30 minutes, and stir halfway through the baking.
4. Sprinkle the granola over the top of the pears and return to the oven. Bake for a further 5 minutes.
5. Remove from the oven and allow to rest for 5 minutes.
6. Serve hot and enjoy.

Serving Suggestion: Serve this with a dollop of low-fat yogurt over the top.
Variation Tip: Feel free to use a sweetener of your choice.
Nutritional Information per Serving:
Calories 201 | Fat 0g | Sodium 7mg | Carbs 38g | Fiber 6g | Sugar 10g | Protein 4g

Grilled Pineapple

Prep Time: 10 minutes
Cook Time: 5 minutes
Serves: 6
Ingredients:
- Vegetable oil
- A pinch of Iodized salt
- 1 pineapple
- 1 tablespoon lime juice extract
- 1 tablespoon olive oil
- 1 tablespoon raw honey
- 3 tablespoons brown sugar

Preparation:
1. Peel the pineapple, remove the eyes of the fruit, and discard the core. Slice lengthwise, forming six wedges. Mix the rest of the fixing in a bowl until blended.
2. Brush the coating mixture on the pineapple (reserve some for basting). Grease an oven or outdoor grill rack with vegetable oil.
3. Place the pineapple wedges on the grill rack and heat for a few minutes per side until golden brownish, basting it frequently with a reserved glaze.
4. Serve on a platter.

Serving Suggestion: Garnish with mint leaves.
Variation Tip: Feel free to omit the iodized salt.
Nutritional Information per Serving:
Calories 97 | Fat 2g | Sodium 2mg | Carbs 20g | Fiber 1g | Sugar 3g | Protein 1g

Stuffed Apples

Prep Time: 5 minutes
Cook Time: 40 minutes
Serves: 2
Ingredients:
- ½ cup oats
- ½ cup pecans, chopped
- 1½ tablespoons unsweetened applesauce
- ½ teaspoon ground cinnamon
- ¼ teaspoon ground ginger
- ¼ teaspoon allspice
- 2 apples
- ½ cup water

Preparation:
1. Preheat the baking oven to 350° F.
2. Meanwhile, add pecans, oats, applesauce and spices in a bowl. Mix well. Set aside.
3. Now, remove the top of each apple and scoop out the flesh from inside.
4. Stuff the apples with the pecan mixture and place them in the baking dish.
5. Add water in the baking dish and place it in the baking oven.
6. Bake for about 40 minutes and take out.
7. Serve and enjoy!

Serving Suggestions: Serve with honey on the top.
Variation Tip: Ground ginger can be omitted.
Nutritional Information per Serving:
Calories: 239 | Fat: 4.3g | Sat Fat: 0.5g | Carbohydrates: 50.7g | Fiber: 8.7g | Sugar: 27.8g | Protein: 3.8g

Frozen Avocado Yogurt

Prep Time: 5 minutes
Serves: 2
Ingredients:
• 1 avocado, peeled and chopped
• ½ teaspoon organic vanilla extract
• 1½ tablespoon powdered stevia
• ¼ cup unsweetened almond milk
• ½ teaspoon fresh mint leaves
• ¼ cup fat-free plain Greek yogurt
• ½ tablespoon fresh lemon juice
Preparation:
1. Add everything except mint leaves in a blender and blend until creamy and smooth.
2. Pour the mixture in an airtight container and freeze for two to three hours.
3. Take out and set aside for about 15 minutes.
4. Top with mint leaves and serve.
Serving Suggestions: Serve with avocado slices on the top.
Variation Tip: Stevia can be omitted.
Nutritional Information per Serving:
Calories: 232 | Fat: 20.1g | Sat Fat: 4.2g | Carbohydrates: 10.4g | Fiber: 6.9g | Sugar: 1.8g | Protein: 5.1g

Frozen Mango Treat

Prep Time: 5 minutes
Serves: 2
Ingredients:
• 1½ cup frozen mangoes, peeled and chopped
• ½ tablespoon fresh mint leaves
• 1 tablespoon fresh lime juice
• ¼ cup chilled water

Preparation: Add all the ingredients in a blender and blend well.
1. Take out and refrigerate for about two hours.
2. Serve and enjoy!
Serving Suggestions: Serve with whipped cream and mango slices on the top.
Variation Tip: You can add honey to enhance taste.
Nutritional Information per Serving:
Calories: 278 | Fat: 1.7g | Sat Fat: 0.4g | Carbohydrates: 69.9g | Fiber: 7.5g | Sugar: 62.4g | Protein: 3.9g

Fruit and Almond Bites

Prep Time: 10 minutes
Cook Time: 35 minutes
Servings: 20
Ingredients:
• 3¾ cups sliced almonds, divided
• ¼ teaspoon almond extract
• ¼ cup honey
• 2 cups dried apricots, finely chopped
• 1 cup dried cherries, finely chopped
• 1 cup pistachios, toasted and finely chopped
Preparation:
1. Pulse 1¼ cups of almonds in a food processor until coarsely chopped. Place the almonds in a shallow dish and set aside for coating.
2. Pulse the remaining 2½ cups of almonds until finely chopped in a food processor. Add the almond extract. Gradually add the honey to the processor while it's running.
3. Transfer the mixture to a large mixing bowl and add the apricots and cherries. Divide the mixture into six equal pieces and roll each into a ½-inch-thick roll. Wrap in plastic wrap and chill for 1 hour.
4. Unwrap and cut the rolls into 1½-inch pieces. Roll half in the reserved almonds, pressing gently to adhere. Pistachio-roll the remaining half.
5. Wrap each one in waxed paper, twisting the ends together to shut them, and store in airtight containers until serving.
6. Serve and enjoy!
Serving Suggestion: Serve with tea.
Variation Tip: You can also add cranberries.
Nutritional Information per Serving:
Calories: 86|Fat: 5g|Sat Fat: 0g|Carbohydrates: 10g|Fiber: 2g|Sugar: 7g|Protein: 2g

Grilled Peaches

Prep Time: 10 minutes
Cook Time: 10 minutes
Serves: 8
Ingredients:
• 4 large peaches, halved and pitted
• ¼ teaspoon ground cinnamon
Preparation:
1. Preheat the grill to medium-high heat and grease the grill grate.
2. Arrange the peaches on grill grate and grill for five minutes per side.
3. Sprinkle with cinnamon and serve.
Serving Suggestions: Serve with honey on the top.
Variation Tip: Some spices can also be added.
Nutritional Information per Serving:
Calories: 30 | Fat: 0.2g | Sat Fat: 0g | Carbohydrates: 7.1g | Fiber: 1.2g | Sugar: 7g | Protein: 0.7g

Peach Sorbet

Prep Time: 5 minutes
Serves: 3
Ingredients:
• 3 peaches, chopped
• 1½ tablespoons unsalted almonds, chopped
• ¼ teaspoon ground cinnamon
• ½ teaspoon organic vanilla extract
• 1 cup unsweetened coconut milk
Preparation:
1. Add peaches in a blender and pulse until a puree is formed.
2. Add in remaining ingredients and pulse until smooth.
3. Pour the mixture in an ice cream maker and process according to maker's directions.
4. Take out and transfer in an airtight container.
5. Freeze for five hours and take out.
6. Serve and enjoy!
Serving Suggestions: Top with peach slices before serving.
Variation Tip: Almonds can be omitted.
Nutritional Information per Serving:
Calories: 309 | Fat: 24.9g | Sat Fat: 17.3g | Carbohydrates: 21g | Fiber: 5.5g | Sugar: 17.2g | Protein: 5.5g

Raspberry Ice cream

Prep Time: 5 minutes
Serves: 3
Ingredients:
• 1½ cup fresh raspberries, divided
• 1 cup unsweetened almond milk
• 5 dates, pitted and chopped
• ½ tablespoon fresh lemon juice
• ½ avocado, peeled and chopped
• ¼ cup unsalted cashews, soaked and drained
• ½ tablespoon fresh beet juice
Preparation:

1. Add ¾ cup raspberries and all the other ingredients in a blender and blend well.
2. Transfer the mixture in an ice cream maker and process according to maker's directions.
3. Transfer the mixture in an airtight container and freeze for four to five hours.
4. Take out and top with remaining raspberries.
5. Serve and enjoy!
Serving Suggestions: Serve with raspberry syrup on the top.
Variation Tip: Coconut milk can also be used.
Nutritional Information per Serving:
Calories: 305 | Fat: 14.5g | Sat Fat: 2.6g | Carbohydrates: 44.8g | Fiber: 18.7g | Sugar: 19.7g | Protein: 5.8g

Raspberry Jelly

Prep Time: 5 minutes
Cook Time: 40 minutes
Serves: 2
Ingredients:
• 2¼ cups fresh raspberries
• 2 tablespoons water
• ½ tablespoon fresh lemon juice
Preparation:
1. Add raspberries and water in a pan and cook for ten minutes on low heat. Stirring occasionally.
2. Add in lemon juice and cook for 30 minutes.
3. Strain the mixture in a bowl and set aside to cool.
4. Transfer it in a blender and blend until jelly like texture is formed.
5. Transfer in serving bowls and refrigerate for one hour before serving.
Serving Suggestions: Serve with raspberry syrup on the top.
Variation Tip: More raspberries can be added.
Nutritional Information per Serving:
Calories: 169 | Fat: 2.1g | Sat Fat: 0.1g | Carbohydrates: 38.6g | Fiber: 21g | Sugar: 14.4g | Protein: 3.9g

Raspberry Mousse

Prep Time: 5 minutes
Serves: 2
Ingredients:
• 1¼ cups fresh raspberries
• ½ teaspoon liquid stevia
• ½ tablespoon fresh lemon juice
• ½ cup unsweetened almond milk

Preparation:
1. Add raspberries, stevia, lemon juice and almond milk in a blender and pulse until smooth.
2. Take out and refrigerate.
3. Serve and enjoy!
Serving Suggestions: Top with raspberries before serving.
Variation Tip: Granulated Erythritol can be added to enhance taste.
Nutritional Information per Serving:
Calories: 99 | Fat: 2g | Sat Fat: 0.1g | Carbohydrates: 20.8g | Fiber: 11.3g | Sugar: 7.6g | Protein: 2.3g

Fruity Bread Pudding

Prep Time: 15 minutes
Cook Time: 50 minutes
Servings: 5
Ingredients:
• 2 tablespoons unsalted margarine, softened
• 1 cup mango, peeled, pitted, and cut into ½-inch pieces
• ½ cup dried apricots, chopped into small pieces
• ½ cup unsalted walnuts, chopped
• ½ teaspoon ground cinnamon
• 6 whole-wheat bread slices
• 1 cup apple, peeled and cut into small pieces
• ½ cup raisins
• 1½ cups fresh apple juice
• ½ teaspoon stevia
Preparation:
1. Preheat the oven to 350°F. Lightly grease a 9-inch x 9-inch baking dish.
2. Lightly spread the margarine over the bread slices.
3. Cut each bread slice into 1-inch pieces. Mix the bread pieces, mangos, apples, apricots, raisins, and walnuts in a large bowl.
4. Mix the apple juice, cinnamon, and stevia in a small bowl. Place the juice mixture over the bread mixture and combine well.
5. Place the mixture into the prepared baking dish evenly and cover with foil.
6. Bake for about 30 minutes. Uncover and bake for about 20 minutes or until the top becomes golden brown.
7. Serve warm and enjoy!
Serving Suggestion: Top with fruit chunks.
Variation Tip: You can use any bread.
Nutritional Information per Serving:
Calories: 320|Fat: 13g|Sat Fat: 2g|Carbohydrates: 46g|Fiber: 5.6g|Sugar: 25g|Protein: 8.1g

Ricotta Mousse

Prep Time: 10 minutes plus 4–6 hours chilling
Servings: 2
Ingredients:
- 1 cup ricotta cheese
- 2 teaspoons cacao powder
- 2 tablespoons fresh blackberries
- 2 teaspoons stevia powder
- ½ teaspoon organic vanilla extract

Preparation:
1. Add all the ingredients except the blackberries to a large bowl and beat until well combined.
2. Transfer the mousse into two serving glasses and refrigerate to chill for about 4–6 hours or until completely set.
3. Serve and enjoy!
Serving Suggestion: Serve with a garnishing of the blackberries.
Variation Tip: You can also add chopped nuts.
Nutritional Information per Serving:
Calories: 182|Fat: 10g|Sat Fat: 4g|Carbohydrates: 8g|Fiber: 1g|Sugar: 1g|Protein: 14g

Apple Crisp

Prep Time: 15 minutes
Cook Time: 20 minutes
Servings: 2
Ingredients:
Filling
- 2 large apples, peeled, cored, and chopped
- 2 tablespoons fresh apple juice
- 2 tablespoons water
- ¼ teaspoon ground cinnamon
Topping
- ½ cup quick rolled oats
- 2 tablespoons unsalted walnuts, chopped
- ¼ cup unsweetened coconut flakes
- ½ teaspoon ground cinnamon
- ¼ cup water

Preparation:
1. Preheat the oven to 300°F. Add all the filling ingredients to a large baking dish and gently mix.
2. Put all the topping ingredients in a mixing bowl and mix until well combined. Spread the topping over the filling mixture evenly.
3. Bake for about 20 minutes or until the top becomes golden brown. Serve warm.
4. Serve and enjoy!
Serving Suggestion: Sprinkle cinnamon on top.
Variation Tip: You can skip the walnuts.
Nutritional Information per Serving:
Calories: 230|Fat: 7g|Sat Fat: 3g|Carbohydrates: 38g|Fiber: 5g|Sugar: 24g|Protein: 3g

Strawberry Crumble

Prep Time: 15 minutes
Cook Time: 25 minutes
Servings: 4
Ingredients:
- 1½ cups fresh strawberries, hulled and chopped
- ½ cup oat flour
- 1½ tablespoons almond butter
- ¼ teaspoon ground cinnamon
- 1 teaspoon arrowroot starch
- 2 tablespoons almond flour
- 2 tablespoons pecans, chopped

Preparation:
1. Preheat the oven to 350°F. For the filling, place the strawberries and arrowroot starch in a baking dish and gently mix.
2. For the topping, add the remaining ingredients to a bowl and mix until a crumbly mixture forms.

3. Spread the topping over the strawberries evenly. Bake for about 20–25 minutes or until the top becomes golden brown.
4. Serve warm and enjoy!
Serving Suggestion: Sprinkle cinnamon on top.
Variation Tip: You can also add more berries.
Nutritional Information per Serving:
Calories: 162|Fat: 9g|Sat Fat: 3g|Carbohydrates: 15g|Fiber: 3.7g|Sugar: 3g|Protein: 3.6g

Dash Brownies

Prep Time: 10 minutes
Cook Time: 30 minutes
Serves: 2
Ingredients:
• 6 ounces dark chocolate, chopped
• 4 egg whites
• ½ cup hot water
• 1 teaspoon vanilla extract
• ⅔ cup coconut sugar
• 1 and ½ cups whole wheat flour
• ½ cup walnuts, chopped
• Cooking spray
• 1 teaspoon baking powder
Preparation:
1. In a bowl, combine the chocolate and the hot water and whisk well. Add vanilla extract and egg whites and whisk well again.
2. In another bowl, combine the sugar with flour, baking powder, and walnuts and stir.
3. Combine the two mixtures, stir well, pour this into a cake pan greased with cooking spray, spread well, bake in the oven for 30 minutes, cool down, slice, and serve.
4. Enjoy!
Serving Suggestion: Serve with a hot beverage.
Variation Tip: Substitute whole wheat flour with almond flour.
Nutritional Information per Serving:
Calories 140 | Fat 10g | Sodium 138mg | Carbs 14g | Fiber1g | Sugar 8g | Protein 2g

Blueberry Orange Compote

Prep Time: 10 minutes

Cook Time: 15 minutes
Serves: 2
Ingredients:
• 5 tablespoons coconut sugar
• 1 ounce orange juice
• 1 pound blueberries
Preparation:
1. In a pot, combine the sugar with the orange juice and blueberries and then toss.
2. Bring to a boil over medium heat, cook for 15 minutes, divide into bowls and serve cold.
3. Enjoy!
Serving Suggestion: Serve with some Greek yogurt and orange slices.
Variation Tip: Substitute orange juice with grapefruit juice.
Nutritional Information per Serving:
Calories 170 | Fat 2g | Sodium 2mg | Carbs 37g | Fiber 2g | Sugar 20g | Protein 0g

Chocolate Tofu Mousse

Prep Time: 10 minutes
Serves: 3
Ingredients:
• ½ pound firm tofu, pressed and drained
• ½ tablespoon organic vanilla extract
• 2 tablespoons unsweetened almond milk
• 1 tablespoon cocoa powder
• 7 drops liquid stevia
Preparation:
1. Add everything in a blender and pulse until smooth and creamy.
2. Take out in serving bowls and refrigerate for two hours.
3. Serve and enjoy!
Serving Suggestions: Serve with chocolate chips on the top.
Variation Tip: You can use chocolate syrup to enhance taste.
Nutritional Information per Serving:
Calories: 65 | Fat: 3.5g | Sat Fat: 0.8g | Carbohydrates: 2.6g | Fiber: 1.3g | Sugar: 0.8g | Protein: 6.6g

Blackberry Crumble

Prep Time: 10 minutes
Cook Time: 40 minutes
Servings: 4
Ingredients:
- ¼ cup coconut flour
- ¾ teaspoon baking soda
- ¼ cup banana, peeled and mashed
- 3 tablespoons water
- ¼ cup arrowroot flour
- 2 tablespoons olive oil
- ½ tablespoons fresh lemon juice
- 1½ cups fresh blackberries

Preparation:
1. Preheat the oven to 300°F. Lightly grease an 8-inch x 8-inch baking dish.
2. In a large bowl, mix all the ingredients except the blackberries.
3. Place the blackberries in the bottom of the prepared baking dish.
4. Spread the flour mixture over the blackberries evenly. Bake for 35–40 minutes or until the top becomes golden brown.
5. Serve warm and enjoy!

Serving Suggestion: Sprinkle lemon juice on top.
Variation Tip: You can also add almonds.
Nutritional Information per Serving:
Calories: 99|Fat: 7g|Sat Fat: 2g|Carbohydrates: 8.9g|Fiber: 3.5g|Sugar: 1.3g|Protein: 10g

Chocolate Cupcakes

Prep Time: 10 minutes
Cook Time: 20 minutes

Servings: 6
Ingredients:
- 1 cup water
- 1 cup oat flour
- 1 tablespoon organic baking powder
- ¼ cup unsweetened almond milk
- 1 cup dates, pitted
- ⅓ cup cacao powder
- Pinch of salt

Preparation:
1. Preheat the oven to 350°F. Line 6 cups of a muffin tin with paper liners.
2. In a food processor, add the water and dates and pulse until smooth.
3. Mix the flour, cacao powder, baking powder, and salt in a large bowl. Add the almond milk and date paste and beat until well combined.
4. Transfer the mixture into the paper muffin cups. Bake in the preheated oven for 25 minutes.
5. Remove the muffin tin from the oven and place it onto a wire rack to cool for about 10 minutes. Carefully invert the cupcakes onto a wire rack to cool completely before serving.
6. Serve and enjoy!

Serving Suggestion: Top with chocolate syrup.
Variation Tip: You can use any milk.
Nutritional Information per Serving:
Calories: 159|Fat: 2.2g|Sat Fat: 1g|Carbohydrates: 26g|Fiber: 5g|Sugar: 18g|Protein: 3.7g

Bean Brownies

Prep Time: 10 minutes
Cook Time: 30 minutes
Servings: 12
Ingredients:
- 2 cups cooked black beans
- 2 tablespoons almond butter
- 2 teaspoons organic vanilla extract
- 1 tablespoon ground cinnamon
- 12 Medjool dates, pitted and chopped
- 2 tablespoons quick rolled oats
- ¼ cup cacao powder

Preparation:
1. Preheat the oven to 350°F. Line a large baking dish with parchment paper.
2. In a food processor, add all the ingredients except the cacao powder and cinnamon and pulse until well combined and smooth.
3. Transfer the mixture into a large bowl. Add the cacao powder and cinnamon and stir to combine. Now, transfer the mixture into the prepared baking dish

evenly and smooth the top surface with the back of a spatula.

4. Bake for about 30 minutes. Remove from the oven and place onto a wire rack to cool completely. With a sharp knife, cut into 12 equal-sized brownies.

5. Serve and enjoy!

Serving Suggestion: Top with chocolate syrup.

Variation Tip: You can also add nuts.

Nutritional Information per Serving:
Calories: 216|Fat: 2.3g|Sat Fat: 1g|Carbohydrates: 42g|Fiber: 8g|Sugar: 18g|Protein: 9g

Pretty Peach Tart

Prep Time: 30 minutes
Cook Time: 40 minutes
Servings: 8
Ingredients:
*   ¼ cup butter, softened
*   2 tablespoons sugar
*   ¼ teaspoon ground nutmeg
*   1 cup all-purpose flour
Filling:
*   2 pounds peaches, peeled and sliced
*   4 tablespoons sugar
*   2 tablespoons all-purpose flour
*   ¼ teaspoon ground cinnamon
*   ¹/₈ teaspoon almond extract
*   ¼ cup sliced almonds
*   Whipped cream, optional

Preparation:
1. Preheat the oven to 375°F.
2. Cream the butter, sugar, and nutmeg until light and creamy. Blend in the flour until it's thoroughly combined.
3. In an ungreased 9-inch fluted tart pan with a removable bottom, press the dough firmly onto the bottom and up the sides.
4. Bake for 10–12 minutes on a medium oven rack until lightly browned. Allow the pastry to cool on a wire rack.
5. To make the filling, toss the peaches with the sugar, flour, cinnamon, and almond extract in a large mixing bowl; pour into the crust. Sprinkle with the almonds.
6. Bake the tart on a lower oven rack for 40–45 minutes, or until the crust is golden brown and the peaches have softened. Allow the tart to cool on a wire rack.
7. Serve and enjoy!

Serving Suggestion: Serve with whipped cream.

Variation Tip: You can use stevia instead of sugar.

Nutritional Information per Serving:
Calories: 222|Fat: 8g|Sat Fat: 4g|Carbohydrates: 36g|Fiber: 3g|Sugar: 15g|Protein: 4g

Strawberry Soufflé

Prep Time: 15 minutes
Cook Time: 12 minutes
Servings: 6
Ingredients:
*   18 ounces fresh strawberries, hulled
*   5 egg whites, divided
*   ¹/₃ cup unsweetened applesauce, divided
*   4 teaspoons fresh lemon juice

Preparation:
1. Preheat the oven to 350°F.
2. In a blender, add the strawberries and pulse until pureed. Strain the mixture into a bowl and discard the seeds.
3. In the same bowl, add 2 egg whites, the lemon juice, and half of the applesauce and beat until frothy and light. In another bowl, add the remaining egg whites and beat until foamy.
4. While beating gradually, add the remaining applesauce and beat until stiff peaks form.
5. Gently fold the egg whites into the strawberry mixture. Transfer the mixture into 6 large ramekins evenly. Arrange the ramekins onto a baking sheet. Bake for about 10–12 minutes.
6. Serve warm and enjoy!

Serving Suggestion: Top with strawberry chunks.

Variation Tip: You can add some vanilla extract.

Nutritional Information per Serving:
Calories: 48|Fat: 0.4g|Sat Fat: 1g|Carbohydrates: 8.3g|Fiber: 1.9g|Sugar: 5.8g|Protein: 3.6g

Avocado Pudding

Prep Time: 10 minutes
Serves: 2
Ingredients:
- 1 cup chopped banana
- ¼ cup fresh lime juice
- 1 avocado, peeled and chopped
- ¼ cup fresh lemon juice
- ½ teaspoon fresh lime zest, finely grated
- ½ teaspoon fresh lemon zest, finely grated
- ½ cup unsweetened applesauce

Preparation:
1. Add everything in a blender and blend until a creamy mixture is formed.
2. Take out and pour in serving glasses.
3. Refrigerate for about three hours, serve and enjoy!

Serving Suggestions: Top with avocado slices before serving.
Variation Tip: Applesauce can be replaced with honey.
Nutritional Information per Serving:
Calories: 307 | Fat: 20.1g | Sat Fat: 4.4g | Carbohydrates: 33.9g | Fiber: 9.6g | Sugar: 16.6g | Protein: 3.1g

Chickpea Fudge

Prep Time: 10 minutes
Cook Time: 5 minutes
Servings: 12
Ingredients:
- 2 cups cooked chickpeas
- ½ cup almond butter
- 1 teaspoon organic vanilla extract
- 8 Medjool dates, pitted and chopped
- ½ cup unsweetened almond milk
- 2 tablespoons cacao powder

Preparation:
1. Line a large baking dish with parchment paper.
2. Add all the ingredients except the cacao powder to a food processor and pulse until well combined.
3. Transfer the mixture to a large bowl and stir in the cacao powder. Transfer the mixture into the prepared baking dish evenly and smooth the top surface with a spatula.
4. Refrigerate for about 2 hours. Cut into desired-sized squares.
5. Serve and enjoy!

Serving Suggestion: Sprinkle cocoa powder on top.
Variation Tip: You can use any milk.
Nutritional Information per Serving:
Calories: 61|Fat: 1.4g|Sat Fat: 1g|Carbohydrates: 10g|Fiber: 2.8g|Sugar: 3.9g|Protein: 2.5g

4-Week Meal Plan

Week 1

Day	Breakfast	Lunch	Snack	Dinner	Dessert
Day 1	Veggie Toasts	Citrus Beef Stir Fry	Rosemary Potato Shells	Salmon Couscous Salad	Walnut Chocolate Chip Cookies
Day 2	Banana Oatmeal Pancakes	Dijon Salmon With Green Bean Pilaf	Roasted Butternut Squash Fries	Poached Salmon with Mustard-Dill Sauce	Raspberry Mousse
Day 3	Mushroom Frittata	Tuna Stuffed Avocados	Baked Cheese Envelopes	Prawns & Veggie Curry	Chocolate Pudding
Day 4	Baked Carrot Oatmeal	Slow-Cooked Mediterranean Chicken and Chickpea Soup	Tomato Basil Bruschetta	Spicy Seafood Stew	Almond and Apricot Biscotti
Day 5	Carrot and Spice Quick Bread	Baked Lamb Meatballs	Basil Pesto Stuffed Mushrooms	Cod & Veggies Bake	Yogurt Cheesecake
Day 6	Quinoa Bread	Tomato & Feta Salad	Basil Tomato Crostini	Spinach and Zucchini Risotto	Chocolate Tofu Mousse
Day 7	Raspberry Smoothie Bowl	Chicken Souvlaki Kabobs With Mediterranean Couscous	Grilled Asparagus	Salmon with Salsa	Strawberry Trifle

Week 2

Day	Breakfast	Lunch	Snack	Dinner	Dessert
Day 1	Buckwheat Pancakes	Chicken Stew	Marinated Portobello Mushrooms with Provolone	Bruschetta Chicken	Sweet Potato and Squash Pie
Day 2	Banana Bread	Asparagus Soup	Kale Chips with Feta	Balsamic Roast Chicken Breast	Avocado Pudding
Day 3	Muesli Breakfast Bars	Chicken and Spring Vegetable Tortellini Salad	Garlicky Green Beans	Healthy Mac and Cheese	Dark Chocolate Kefir Parfait
Day 4	Green Smoothie Bowl	Roasted Pork Loin and Potatoes	Pickled Eggs	Chicken and Broccoli Stir-Fry	Strawberries and Cream Cheese Crepes
Day 5	Cherry Pancakes	Chicken Lettuce Wraps	Roasted Carrots and Beets	Quinoa Power Salad	Fruit and Almond Bites
Day 6	Zucchini Bread	Grilled Flank Steak with Peach Compote	Cilantro Rice	Turkey Burger	Apple-Berry Cobbler
Day 7	Yogurt and Granola Bowl	Creamy Lemon Pasta with Shrimp	Lemony Zucchini	Chicken & Strawberry Salad	Mocha Chocolate Mousse

Week 3

Day	Breakfast	Lunch	Snack	Dinner	Dessert
Day 1	Apple Crepes	Spicy Bean Chili	Chili-Lime Grilled Pineapple	Southwestern Vegetable Tacos	Pretty Peach Tart
Day 2	Whole-Wheat Soda Bread	Roasted Vegetables with Cheese Polenta	Lemony Mushrooms	Slow-Cooked Mediterranean Chicken and Orzo	Baked Apples with Cherries and Almonds
Day 3	Eggs on Toast	Mediterranean Chickpea Quinoa Bowl	Garlicky Carrots	Zucchini Pepper Kebabs	Ricotta Mousse
Day 4	Pear-Cauliflower Porridge	Cheesy Pasta Bake	Mashed Sweet Potatoes	Baked Chicken and Wild Rice	Delicious Fudge
Day 5	Spiced Carrot and Raisin Tea Bread	Eggplant Parmesan	Sausage-Stuffed Zucchini	Turkey Stir Fry with Vegetables	Fruit Cake
Day 6	Chickpea Polenta with Olives	Cherry Chicken Wraps	Lemony Kale & Carrot	Pasta & Beans Stew	Apple Crisp
Day 7	Apple Porridge	Sweet and Sour Cabbage with Pork Chops	Brown-Rice Pilaf	Chicken & Broccoli Casserole	Lime Cherry Cream

Week 4

Day	Breakfast	Lunch	Snack	Dinner	Dessert
Day 1	French Toast	Quinoa Bowl	Spicy Almonds	Roasted Lemon Swordfish	Carrot Cake Cookies
Day 2	Omelet Waffles	Fajita Chili	Pickled Asparagus	Roasted Salmon With Smoky Chickpeas and Greens	Cashew Cream Mousse
Day 3	Whole-Grain Pancakes	Cajun Baked Trout	Cannellini Bean Hummus	Mixed Vegetarian Chili	Strawberry Crumble
Day 4	Cranberry Orange Muffins	Crusted Salmon	Zucchini Sticks	Gnocchi Pomodoro	Cinnamon Applesauce
Day 5	Wheat Berries and Fruits Bowl	Linguini Chicken Soup	Broccoli with Bell Peppers	Chicken Tikka	Vanilla Poached Peaches
Day 6	Apple Omelet	Veggie Pita Rolls	Portobello Mushroom Florentine	Slow-Cooked Pasta e Fagioli Soup	Blackberry Crumble
Day 7	Quinoa Porridge	Chicken and Vegetable Penne Pasta	Butternut Squash Fries	Pumpkin Rice	Fig Bars

The introduction of this book examined different aspects of the Dash Diet. It explained the diet's origins, health benefits, relationships with various conditions, and the studies that led to its formation. This book provides a basic explanation of the Dash Diet to its readers.

In addition to all of this useful knowledge, the final chapters include numerous tasty Dash recipes. A 28-day healthy meal plan is also included to assist beginners in getting their DASH regimen off to a better start. Are you ready to counter hypertension through a dietary change? Well, this book will help you get started on your journey to a healthier you.

Good luck and enjoy the delicious meals that await you!

VOLUME EQUIVALENTS(DRY)

US STANDARD	METRIC (APPROXIMATE)
1/8 teaspoon	0.5 mL
1/4 teaspoon	1 mL
1/2 teaspoon	2 mL
3/4 teaspoon	4 mL
1 teaspoon	5 mL
1 tablespoon	15 mL
1/4 cup	59 mL
1/2 cup	118 mL
3/4 cup	177 mL
1 cup	235 mL
2 cups	475 mL
3 cups	700 mL
4 cups	1 L

VOLUME EQUIVALENTS(LIQUID)

US STANDARD	US STANDARD (OUNCES)	METRIC (APPROXIMATE)
2 tablespoons	1 fl.oz.	30 mL
1/4 cup	2 fl.oz.	60 mL
1/2 cup	4 fl.oz.	120 mL
1 cup	8 fl.oz.	240 mL
1 1/2 cup	12 fl.oz.	355 mL
2 cups or 1 pint	16 fl.oz.	475 mL
4 cups or 1 quart	32 fl.oz.	1 L
1 gallon	128 fl.oz.	4 L

WEIGHT EQUIVALENTS

US STANDARD	METRIC (APPROXIMATE)
1 ounce	28 g
2 ounces	57 g
5 ounces	142 g
10 ounces	284 g
15 ounces	425 g
16 ounces (1 pound)	455 g
1.5 pounds	680 g
2 pounds	907 g

TEMPERATURES EQUIVALENTS

FAHRENHEIT(F)	CELSIUS(C) (APPROXIMATE)
225 °F	107 °C
250 °F	120 °C
275 °F	135 °C
300 °F	150 °C
325 °F	160 °C
350 °F	180 °C
375 °F	190 °C
400 °F	205 °C
425 °F	220 °C
450 °F	235 °C
475 °F	245 °C
500 °F	260 °C

Additional Considerations for Modular DCS Layouts

Modular layouts are generally wired using buss type wiring where Hot and Common wires travel around the layout and connect to themselves as a pair of circles, or an electrical buss. This generally precludes any attempt at using the aforementioned track block and terminal block concepts inherent in star or home run wiring.

Instead, DCS should be added as discussed previously in Adding DCS to an Existing Layout. Where necessary, signal strength may be improved by placing 18 volt light bulbs across the buss wiring of Hot and Common wires that run beneath the modules.

Part IV - Introduction to DCS WiFi

1. What is WiFi?

WiFi is the popular name for a networking standard designated as "802.11" by a standards committee of the IEEE (Institute of Electrical and Electronics Engineers). This standard is used to implement wireless local area networks (LANs) that allow computers and other devices to communicate with each other. While this definition isn't all that important for the purposes of DCS, what WiFi does most certainly is. It's what allows a smart phone or WiFi-enabled tablet to communicate with DCS. WiFi is what allows the DCS Application to operate engines, accessories and switch tracks.

2. Overview of DCS WiFi Operation

To properly understand WiFi's role in providing for DCS Application operation, it is necessary to discuss the actual requirements of a WiFi network for a DCS layout and also the process of communication between the DCS Application and DCS engines.

WiFi Network Requirements

There are two methods you can use to establish a WiFi network for a DCS layout:

- The first method uses an already present home WiFi network. The DCS WiFi Interface Unit (WIU) is wirelessly connected to the existing home network. It is then accessible from the DCS Application installed on the smart device by simply connecting the smart device to the existing WiFi network.
- The second method is by using the network that is built-into the MTH WIU itself. The smart device then is connected directly to the WiFi network generated by the WIU.

These two connection methods are explained in detail later in this book.

Communication Between the DCS Application, WIU, TIU, and DCS Engines

The DCS Application and the WIU engage in wireless two-way communication using WiFi. The WIU and TIU engage in two-way communication using the WIU's USB port, and the TIU's USB port (Rev. L TIU or later) or the TIU's serial port. TIUs and DCS engines engage in two-way communication by sending data packets through the rails.

In general, the sequence of events when you want to send a command to a DCS engine is as follows:

- Tap a key on the DCS Application to instruct a DCS engine to do something, such as ringing the bell, sounding the horn, changing direction, turning smoke on or off, etc.
- The DCS Application causes the smart device to send a WiFi command to the WIU.
- The WIU forwards that command over a wire to the TIU.
- The TIU determines for which DCS engine the command is intended and sends data packets through the rails to that engine.
- The engine receives the data packets, sends acknowledgement data packets through the rails back to the TIU and executes the command.
- The TIU sends an acknowledgement to the WIU, which wirelessly forwards the acknowledgement back to the DCS Application on the smart device, indicating that the DCS engine has acknowledged the command.
- This communication process is depicted below, in Figure 2 - Packet Flow Diagram.